BETTER SLEEP FOR THE OVERACHIEVER

FOREWORD BY MICHAEL BREUS

ANNE BARTOLUCCI

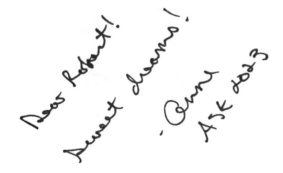

AIBHS

ABOUT BETTER SLEEP FOR THE OVERACHIEVER

Does your inner drive keep you up all night? Discover methods to ease your ambitious mind into a healthy, highly productive pattern of sleep.

Do you toss and turn worrying about tomorrow's to-do list? Does your body crave rest but your brain won't shut down? Have you tried all the recommended bedtime tricks and found no relief? Insomnia specialist and clinical psychologist Anne D. Bartolucci, Ph.D. has spent more than a decade helping results-driven people catch some z's. Now this fellow overachiever is here to show you a simple way to get the restorative repose you need to fuel your busy lifestyle.

Better Sleep for the Overachiever is a thorough guide to creating a lifelong habit of healthy, rejuvenating slumber patterns to help you perform at your peak. Drawing on Bartolucci's extensive experience, you'll discover why insomnia isn't just a nighttime problem—it's deeply intertwined with your daily thoughts and activities. Using simple strategies to identify and defuse stressful behaviors, you'll soon be drifting off to dreamland!

In *Better Sleep for the Overachiever*, you'll discover:
- Step-by-step tips and best practices to wind down in the evening
- Why perfectionism and imposter syndrome stifle quality sleep and how to overcome them
- The time management skills needed to let go and allow your mind to settle
- An exploration of the role that mindfulness plays in managing racing thoughts
- Real-life case studies, conversations from Bartolucci's practice, and much, much more!

Better Sleep for the Overachiever is an easily accessible handbook to help you snooze like a pro. If you like expert advice, practical techniques, and proven research, then you'll love Anne D. Bartolucci's life-changing resource.

Buy *Better Sleep for the Overachiever* to get the rest you deserve tonight!

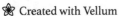

ACKNOWLEDGEMENTS

As you can probably imagine, this type of book is an undertaking of passion, and such projects do best when the author has had a lot of support. I'm lucky to be one of those authors.

First and foremost, I'd like to thank my patients. I used to be annoyed when fellow therapists would only want to refer to other therapists who had a certain amount of experience. Then, the longer I was in practice, I came to realize that I've learned so much from the people who allow me to help them, probably even more than I learned during my training now that I'm more than a decade out of school. My patients also opened my eyes to the overachiever personality type and inspired me to write this book. So, if you're one of them, thank you. You have taught me so much, and I'm honored to have been part of your journey.

Second, I definitely need to acknowledge the support of my husband Jason. He keeps me grounded when I'm going in a thousand different directions. He also encourages me to be the best version of myself.

Next, thank you to my colleague and fellow sleep psychologist Jackie Kloss, Ph.D., C.B.S.M., and fellow Decaturite and overachiever Brennen Dicker, Executive Director of the Creative Media Industries Institute at Georgia State, for being my beta readers and for your valuable feedback. I'd also like to thank my editor Kerry Higgens Wendt for her patience as I struggled through many of the things I wrote about, especially the procrastination parts.

Last and definitely not least, BIG thanks to my mentor and friend Michael Breus, Ph.D., D.A.B.S.M., who first trained me in sleep and who wrote the foreword for this book. Mike, thank you for your guidance and encouragement at every step of my career.

FOREWORD
MICHAEL BREUS, PH.D., D.A.B.S.M.

I was excited to read *Better Sleep for the OverAchiever*, and even more excited to be able to recommend it to my overachieving patients! In the book, Dr. Bartolucci identifies one of the most difficult patients to treat, by helping us all understand who that person is at their core. She correctly identifies that over-achievers may not respond well to traditional treatments for insomnia and helps us all understand why: difficulty with relaxation, racing thoughts, perfectionism, time management, dealing with failure, and of course procrastination.

While many of these issues can plague us all, the person who is correctly identified as an Overachiever with sleep issues, will need personalized recommendations; and that is exactly what Dr. Bartolucci gives her readers and so much more. All the chapters are referenced and science-based, but there are also many times where Dr. B. shares stories about people she has worked with, where many of us can identify, and learn more. She also summarizes all the important points at the end of each chapter to help the reader review and take action right away. Even after having 20 years of experience with this patient population, I found myself thinking about better ways to deal with many of these issues, based on her work. If you are an insomniac, an overachiever, or someone who wants to get the most out of their sleep, this is the book for you.

Michael Breus PhD is a Board certified Sleep Specialist living in Manhattan Beach CA. Author of three bestselling books, Good Night: The Sleep Doctors 4-week program to Better Sleep and Better Health, The Sleep Doctor's Diet Plan: Lose Weight Through Better Sleep, The Power of When: Discover your Chronotype.

Dr. Breus appears regularly on The Dr. Oz Show, CNN, The Doctors, CBS This Morning and Huffington Post Live. He contributes to The Huffington Post, Psychology Today, and The Dr Oz Blogs.

INTRODUCTION

In 2013, I was invited to participate in the FOCUS conference, which is geared toward non-doctoral level sleep and respiratory specialists. I would travel to Nashville to deliver a talk on something like, "Sleep Tips for the Sleep Professional," and it would theoretically cover much of what I talk to my patients about daily.

Then it occurred to me – why would I want to travel several hours away to give a talk similar to the conversations I have every single day? Plus, why would the audience want to hear the same sleep recommendations they'd heard a hundred times, especially since many of them were in the industry? There's a big difference between talking to someone one-on-one, when you can tailor the conversation to their specific problem, and lecturing on general principles to a large group. The former is interesting and engaging. As for the latter, well, I was afraid I would bore both them and myself. So I came up with a twist: I decided to tailor the talk to a certain kind of patient I see repeatedly.

I've labeled these particular insomnia patients the overachievers. I haven't developed an assessment tool for this yet since my clinical work keeps me busy, but this personality type has appeared often enough that I've seen a pattern emerge. In fact, one of the reasons I wrote this book is because of the response I got when I put the slide deck from the FOCUS presentation in my office. I thought some of my patients might find it interesting to flip through while they waited for their appointments. I've been surprised at how many patients ask me for copies of the presentation because they see so much of themselves in it.

Overachievers can't sleep because their minds race, which is a common complaint. Beyond that, they have a strong sense of drive, they can't relax, and they have trouble letting go of mistakes. Sometimes their minds pounce on them as soon as they get into bed. Other times, they are so exhausted that they fall asleep at the beginning of the night, then – as soon as they've slept enough to start to satisfy their sleep need – they have a normal awakening, and their minds are waiting for them. Even if they're not thinking of stressful topics, the to-do list and other things pop in. I have a certain sympathy for this personality type because I am one.

Yes, my name is Anne, and I am an overachiever. But I sleep very well.

Admittedly, I don't feel very "accomplished" or any of the other terms we overachievers tend to hear. I'm currently experiencing unpredictability in many aspects of my professional life, which is tough for this self-affirmed control freak. Plus, I'm dealing with my own life-script change – more about that later. But in spite of all this uncertainty, I sleep great, at least seven-and-a-half to eight hours a night during the week, and longer on weekends, if I give myself the opportunity.

Unpredictability and uncertainty are parts of life, no matter what we do to avoid them. The same goes for performances and tasks that go less than perfectly, or that we think we've messed up. The mind likes to go over and over and over these small – or large – incidents, often – you guessed it – at night when we're trying to sleep. The good news is that there are ways to work around this tendency and minimize its effects.

In this book, I'm going to go beyond the usual advice you've heard about how to sleep better, although there will be some of that. Hopefully, though, it's presented in a way you'll connect with. I'll share with you some of the tools my overachiever patients – and, to be honest, I myself – have found to be successful. I encourage you to read with an open mind, because your brain may want to dismiss some of what I have to say as stuff you've heard before. But I suspect you'll find new strategies that will help you not only sleep better but also be a more productive person. And who knows? Maybe you'll be happier overall.

If there's no other reason to read this book, keep this in mind: the negative effects of sleeplessness on the brain and body are well-established, and one area that suffers is productivity. If you're an overachiever, you measure yourself against what you can accomplish. It's much easier to meet *your* goals if your brain isn't scrambled by lack of sleep. *My* goal is to help you do just that.

YOU KNOW YOU'RE AN OVERACHIEVER IF

Think back to when you first noticed the need to achieve. There likely wasn't any first step or accomplishment that you remember the way an addict does their first hit. Rather, you had a drive that was always present. Maybe you were a people-pleaser and thrived on others' smiles, laughter, and approval. Perhaps you were a straight-A student who was rewarded for bringing home good grades. Or you might have been the athlete who succeeded on the playing field or pitch to the admiration of your school's fans and coaches.

Or, dare I say, all of the above. It doesn't matter what you were good at; the commonality is that you had the drive to succeed, and you likely gravitated toward areas and activities where your natural talents and abilities made that possible.

Bless your heart.

Oh, I'm sorry. Did I shock you with this Southernism? Let's switch gears, then, and look at the downside of this personality type.

When was your first failure? Or second? Third? I'm guessing you remember these more vividly than you do your early successes. You might still beat yourself up over them. I remember one of mine: I was a freshman in high school, and I was in the required typing course. This being the early nineties, we used typewriters, and there was no convenient backspace key like the one I just used when I adjusted this sentence. I got a C on a test due to the number of mistakes I'd made in typing an assigned line of text, and I was furious. I'd always been a straight-A student. How dare the teacher give me a C?

In truth, this failure challenged my identity. I'd defined myself as a straight-A student, and that C made me anxious and uncertain. After my mother pointed out that I got the grade I deserved for my work, I tried harder. I practiced – excessively – became an excellent typist, and eventually got an A in the class. This was the first of many high-school A's, and eventually I became the class valedictorian. Thus the process of anxiety-driven excessive effort was reinforced. And then in college it was reinforced again. I only got two B's, both in classes where I bumped up against the limits of my own abilities (piano lessons and sight-singing/ear training if you're wondering), and I graduated magna cum laude. It wasn't until years later that I recognized those B's as my most valuable grades, because I'd reached my limitations, and not excelling in those areas was okay. I wasn't perfect at something, and the world didn't end. But for a long time, I wished I had stuck to my major subject areas of mathematics and psychology.

Think about your own career path. Overachievers start out with a goal in mind and tend to follow the next logical step and achievement until we get to a point where we've gotten as far as our talents and abilities will take us. Even better, our natural drive keeps us going, helps us overcome obstacles, and sometimes helps us find creative ways around our limitations. Anxiety gets a bad reputation, but think about it – could you have achieved as much as you did without some level of anxiety?

But what happens to that drive when we reach a point

where we've gotten as far as we can go, or when our next achievement is something far-off like retirement? Even worse, what happens at retirement, when the goals become undefined? I call the former the new midlife crisis, and I've seen it repeatedly with my achievement-driven insomnia patients in their late thirties to mid-forties. The latter, the retirees, have trouble finding their new identity in their transition. No matter what the age, whether it's on a broad stage like life or on a small one like in bed at night, it's hard to stop and let go of the anxiety and drive that's been adaptive and helpful most of your life. When that anxiety has nowhere to go and nothing to apply itself to, it causes problems, including insomnia.

THE IDEA of the overachiever personality type is not new. In 2007, Moneywatch published an article through CBS called *How to Manage Overachievers*, which extolled the advantages of this type of employee but also discussed their limitations. While overachievers are often creative, intelligent, and reliable, they can also be overly tough on themselves or others, impatient when having to deal with others, and extreme in their thinking. They also don't like working on teams, and I suspect I know the reason. Remember group projects in high school or college? How many overachievers ended up doing most of the work and carried the rest of the group along to ensure they'd get an A? Also, while overachievers like to be challenged in their work, they typically don't like their ideas to be challenged by others.

In his 2011 book, *Flying without a Net: Turning Fear of Change into Fuel for Success*[1], Harvard professor Thomas Delong identified eleven characteristics of the "high-need-for-achievement personality." Let's break these characteristics down into some questions. If you're reading on paper, feel free to put a checkmark by the questions you can answer "yes" to. If you're reading a library book or electronically, please don't write on your screen, but keep a running count somewhere. Yes, I know the latter seems like a no-brainer, but I'm assuming you're operating under a certain level of sleep deprivation, which impairs good decision-making like alcohol does.

Please remember that this isn't an empirically validated diagnostic tool with established reliability, but rather an exercise to help you start thinking about your own personality and where it fits within the overachiever type. All insomniacs are different, and most overachievers are, too.

Work style, task achievement drive, and persistent thoughts about getting something done

Do you get a thrill when you achieve something?

Are you motivated by setting goals?

Do you feel that not meeting goals means you've failed?

Are you very afraid of failure?

Is it difficult for you to turn off work when you get home?

Do you check emails right up until bedtime and prioritize work tasks over sleep, especially when you're up against a deadline?

Do you have trouble winding down or relaxing?

Do you often feel that you're not doing enough or that you should be doing something else?

Do you like being busy?

Do you prefer to choose your own projects over having someone else assign them?

Do you like working for yourself (if applicable) or prefer to have more independence and autonomy in your job?

Difficulty prioritizing and perfectionism

Do you procrastinate important tasks or find yourself struggling to meet deadlines due to having put them off?

Do you try to get all the little things out of the way first before you tackle the important ones, and then end up with not enough time for the big things?

When you look at your to-do list, do you get overwhelmed by the sheer volume of tasks?

Do you often find that you're moving too slowly because you're not able to accept that something is complete when it's good enough?

Did you just cringe when you read the phrase *good enough*?

Do you often take on extra challenges even if you're not sure you have time for them?

Do you have trouble saying no?

When you meet goals, do you then set bigger ones even if you said you'd stop with the previous goal (e.g., not only getting all A's but perfect scores on your exams)?

Interpersonal challenges

Is it hard for you to have potentially confrontational conversations with others?

Do you end up doing so in your head to an excessive degree?

Do you often try to guess what others are thinking about you?

Do you feel that you come up lacking no matter how much you accomplish?

Do you have trouble delegating because you don't trust others to do the tasks you assign them or you're concerned they won't perform as well as you would have?

When someone gives you negative feedback, do you obsess over it?

Do you tend to dismiss positive feedback?

Overachiever history

When you were in school, did the adults around you describe you as a "self-starter" or some other term that implied high motivation to initiate tasks or to go beyond what was asked of you?

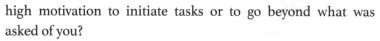 Did you excel in more than one area?

Did you take on extra responsibilities in addition to school and extracurricular activities?

Did adults see you as very reliable and responsible?

Did you start your own business at a young age, or did you want to?

Did you (and do you) have trouble with nitpicky details and processes you don't see a good reason for?

Did advisers ever accuse you of having an aversion to spare time?

MANY PEOPLE WON'T ANSWER yes to every question, but if you checked several of them, you may be an overachiever.

By this point, you're probably wondering what all this has to do with insomnia, although I'm guessing that you're starting to see the connection. I've drawn a lot of these questions from the characteristics of overachievers given in the sources I've mentioned, but I've also drawn them from my patients who have trouble "turning it off," relaxing and letting go of the day. When I talk to them about what keeps them from sleeping, I sometimes frame the overachiever drive as a momentum that we carry through the day. It helps us get things done, but then it runs away with us at night.

Our minds also try to fool us into thinking we don't need to sleep. Have you ever said – or heard anyone say – "I'll sleep when I'm dead?" That phrase reflects a pernicious belief that sleep is a waste of precious time that could be spent doing other, more productive activities. Some overachievers, rather than being caught in the momentum of the day, may want to sleep, but have trained themselves to resist it. Or perhaps they "fight sleep" because their minds don't want to let go of the day.

But then what happens? When they try to sleep, they either can't because they've trained themselves too well, or they get poor-quality sleep and wake feeling unrefreshed. You know how well that works out for productivity.

Another pitfall I've seen frequently is the "one more thing" trap. Someone may have every intention of going to bed at a reasonable hour, but they get caught up in household or work tasks – "I'll just do this one more thing" – and suddenly it's 1:00 a.m. Then they scramble to bed and lie there trying to force themselves to fall asleep quickly because the alarm will go off in a few hours. As we all know, the harder you try to force sleep, the less likely it will happen.

Why do we do this to ourselves? In the next chapter, I'll explain more about how certain personality factors can drive these behaviors and influence sleep.

2

WHY IS THIS HAPPENING TO ME?

M any of my patients have had sleep problems since childhood, but several others have developed insomnia due to various stressors or, in about 10–20 percent of cases, spontaneously and gradually over time. Some of these insomniacs have a family history of insomnia, and others are the sole sufferers in their families, as far as they know at least.

Why people develop insomnia is one of the mysteries of the disorder, although we do find out more as research in the area progresses. Is being a good sleeper or a bad sleeper genetic? Are certain people doomed to develop a pattern of sleepless nights? If there is a biological basis, does that mean the patient is destined for a lifetime of hopping from one sleep aid to another as they develop tolerance and have to switch?

The answer to all of the above questions is not necessarily, and that's one reason I'm writing this book. I want to give you hope. But first I'd like to give you some answers.

. . .

In 1987, Art Spielman and his colleagues proposed what's known as the three-factor model of insomnia development.[1] First, everyone has a certain amount of predisposition to or likelihood of developing the disorder. Think about two people, person A and person B. Person A has a higher predisposition to develop insomnia than person B does. This means that while person A and person B are both sleeping well currently, the same stressor might push person A over the threshold of insomnia development, while person B, who has a lower predisposition, may not develop sleep problems. Do you know someone who sleeps well even though they have a similar level of stress as you? They likely have a lower predisposition to developing insomnia than you do. Another example of differing predisposition is that I see several patients whose spouses sleep very well, despite the fact that they've both gone through the same rough times. While people also handle stress differently – I'll get to that in a bit – the individuals in these couples likely have differing predisposition levels.

Second are the precipitating factors, or the events and stressors that push someone over the threshold and cause them to develop the insomnia. Finally, perpetuating factors, or what keeps the disorder going, are the third factor. We'll talk more about the third factor in later chapters, but for now, we'll focus on what predisposes overachievers to develop sleep problems and what can push them over that edge – for example, how we think and feel about stressors, how we cope with life in general, and, as mentioned above, genetics, which can feed into a predisposition to develop insomnia.

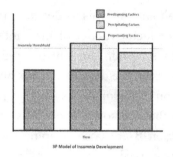

3P Model of Insomnia Development

Personality

As I mentioned previously, once I had been doing insomnia work, I came to recognize a certain personality pattern, which I dubbed the overachiever, common to many of my patients. By definition, personality is a trait that has been present for most of a person's life, starting in childhood. Many of my clients tell me they've had a high need to achieve from an early age. Researchers have been looking into personality using a system called the five-factor model for decades – yes, psychologists like factors – and some have investigated which of these traits apply to insomniacs. First, let's talk about what the five factors are. These definitions are very simplified, but you should get an idea of what they mean:

Neuroticism: the tendency to experience negative emotions

Extraversion: how social someone is and how much they enjoy being in the company of other people

Openness to experience: willingness to try new things

Agreeableness: how well someone gets along with others

Conscientiousness: a measure of self-direction; has the highest overlap with need to achieve[2]

TYPICALLY, when psychologists look at the five-factor model, they consider those who are low on neuroticism and high on the other four factors – extraversion, openness to experience, agreeableness, and conscientiousness – to be more healthy than those on the opposite end of the spectrum. Indeed, as would be expected, individuals low on neuroticism and high on conscientiousness report more sleep, although the highly conscientious ones may also be more likely to sleep lightly.[3]

Individuals with similar traits may differ in their sleep – I certainly see that in my practice, and it keeps me on my toes that every insomniac is different – so it's important to look at the whole picture and across cultures to see if these patterns endure. In the case of insomnia, they do. For example, a study of young women in Korea found that neuroticism negatively correlated with sleep quality, and extraversion, agreeableness, and conscientiousness were all positively associated with it.[4] Another study, of populations in Australia and Finland, found that conscientiousness was not associated with total sleep time, but it did correlate with sleep quality. These researchers made an interesting point that getting better sleep could lead to more agreeableness and conscientiousness, because people who sleep well feel better emotionally and are more motivated to complete tasks.[5] That brings up an interesting point. Many times, sleep problems are considered to be secondary to psychopathology and other situations or traits, but often the relationship is bidirectional. This means that not sleeping causes people to feel worse mentally.

The association between conscientiousness and good sleep presents a problem, because overachievers are notoriously conscientious to a fault, perhaps sometimes at the cost of all else. Not surprisingly, it's been proposed that overly high levels of certain "positive" personality traits can still be maladaptive.[6] For example, being conscientious is supposedly good and is associated with higher measures of work and school success, as well as with sleep, as described above. But at the extreme, being too conscientious has been found to lead to trouble letting go of control, workaholism, preoccupation with rules, difficulty taking risks and making decisions, trouble relying on others, and not being able to deal with loss or failure. Sound familiar? These are similar to and overlap with the traits of DeLong's high-need-for-achievement personality. I see them in many of my patients, who are also highly anxious about their sleep. They ruminate about it during the day, and they focus too much on what they should and shouldn't do before bed, which perpetuates the problem. In fact, sleep often becomes another target of their perfectionism, another personality trait associated with insomnia along with the need for control, a high concern with internal and bodily states, and the tendency to internalize rather than express negative feelings.[7]

With regard to psychopathology, it's well established that insomnia overlaps with anxiety disorders and depression. I have also observed that many of my overachiever patients share symptoms that are characteristic of Obsessive-Compulsive Personality Disorder, or OCPD. The defining parts of this disorder are rigidity around routines and space organization and a high need for control. This disorder differs from Obsessive Compulsive Disorder (OCD) in that, while intrusive thoughts and rigid routines can be present, OCPD lacks the true obsessions and compulsions of OCD.[8]

When personality disorders have been assessed in insomnia patients, OCPD and closely related personality disorders have been found to be associated with poor sleep. In one study, features of OCPD and another personality disorder in the same cluster, Avoidant Personality Disorder, were associated with how much adults who were dependent on hypnotic medication felt their sleep problems negatively affected their functioning during the day and how high their reported levels of tiredness were.[9] In another study, perimenopausal women who suffered from insomnia were more likely to have OCPD than their counterparts without insomnia were.[10] They also scored higher on neuroticism and lower on agreeableness.

When we talk about personality traits and disorders, it's tempting to move in the direction of self-diagnosis, but I urge you to exercise caution. Only a mental health professional can determine, through an interview and other assessment measures, whether you have a personality disorder. According to the current version of the *Diagnostic and Statistical Manual*, the prevalence of OCPD is only 2.1 to 7.9 percent, so it's unlikely you warrant a diagnosis. Also, the core definition of a personality disorder is a lifelong pattern of maladaptive functioning, whereas for overachievers, their drive, anxiety, and perfectionism have been helpful *to a certain point*.

Nonetheless, you may find that some of these descriptions sound a bit too familiar. If you have a personality type that fits the profile – high on neuroticism but low on extraversion, openness to experience, or agreeableness – it may be contributing to some of your sleep problems. As for conscientiousness, we've discussed how this double-edged sword can be helpful but can also encourage the overachiever to focus too much on sleep. Interestingly, it's been found that using sleep-tracking devices, rather than being helpful, can increase the likelihood for insomnia for some patients. Indeed, I've observed that in my practice as well: people become overly concerned with what their devices are telling them and discount their own perceptions.

Hyperarousal

As mentioned, one trait of those who are highly overconscientious is trouble with letting go of control, which is necessary for relaxing and winding down. This sense of physical energy or activation has a name: hyperarousal.

Like personality, hyperarousal has been proposed to be a

trait, or at least a long-term behavioral tendency.[11] Hyper-arousal is also an overachiever personality trait, possibly reflected in the drive to accomplish tasks and goals, or in a sense of drive and energy in general. When I'm in the middle of a busy day or week and stop for a moment to check in with how I feel, it's almost like I can feel a little motor in my chest pushing me to do more, achieve more. If I don't wind down well at night, it keeps my mind racing and can even make it hard to settle down and be physically comfortable.

When researchers have looked at characteristics associated with insomnia, hyperarousal comes up frequently. It has been studied for several decades. Simply put, people with hyper-arousal react more strongly to stressors than those with low arousal do, and they carry emotions with them longer. This can affect how well they handle stress, which can, of course, precip-itate insomnia episodes.

Remember how predisposing factors like personality and hyperarousal push someone closer to the insomnia threshold? One study found that hyperarousal, which they term *arous-ability*, makes someone more likely to develop insomnia in response to stressors. Indeed, they claim it's the "most specific feature of individuals vulnerable to transient insomnia," and they related it to the personality factor of neuroticism.[12] Another study found similar results for those with longer-term insomnia.[13]

One key feature of those with hyperarousal is that since negative emotions happen more easily and stick around longer, stressful events affect them more. This brings us into the realm of precipitating factors, or those events that push someone over the edge to develop insomnia.

Stress Perception and Coping Styles

As for precipitating factors, it's not only what happens but how people react that determines whether they will develop insomnia. Precipitating factors that push an overachiever over the threshold to insomnia could be setbacks, perceived failures, an opportunity to shine (with the extra pressure that comes with it), the advancement or achievement of a colleague or rival, and a life adjustment that includes loss of control. Retirement is a big example of such a transition for many reasons. Difficulty coping with stress has been found to be a precipitating factor for insomnia development, both generally and in peri-menopausal women in particular.[14]

What does unhealthy coping look like? The studies cited above, about temporary and chronic insomnia, also found that when people engage in emotion-oriented coping, they handle stress less well, which leads to sleep problems. Emotion-oriented coping focuses on the emotional impact of the stressor rather than the problem itself.[15] In other words, rather than solving the problem, someone who uses emotion-oriented coping engages in strategies such as stress-eating that will reduce the negative feelings that the problem causes.

But, you may argue, *I have sleep problems because my life is more stressful than the lives of those around me.* Not necessarily. Charles Morin, who wrote the insomnia treatment manual I still use, and his group found that good sleepers and poor sleepers have the same number of stressors. Poor sleepers rated their events as more stressful, and they felt their lives had more uncertainty – and that they had less control over it – than the good sleepers. As you can imagine, this led to more arousal, both physical and mental, at bedtime. They also went for the emotion-focused coping strategies rather than the problem-solving ones. Emotion-focused coping and higher arousability in response to stressors has been shown to be associated with the development of insomnia in other studies as well.[16]

Sometimes problems can't be solved right away, so then what do you do? Starting in the next chapter, I'll give you ideas for how to better deal with stress and to train yourself to not carry so much of the day into the bed with you.

Important Takeaways

- There are three parts to why we develop insomnia – the characteristics that make us likely to develop it, the event that pushes us over the edge, and the thoughts, behaviors, and feelings that keep it going.
- When thinking about personality, it can be helpful to consider where we fall across the five factors of neurotocism, extraversion, openness to experience, agreeableness, and conscientiousness. Conscientiousness has been associated with both better and poor sleep.
- Obsessive-compulsive personality disorder, or OCPD, has been associated with insomnia, but please don't diagnose yourself. Instead, think of the characteristics of this disorder that could be contributing to sleep problems.
- Hyperarousal, or a higher level of perceived physical and mental energy, can make it harder to sleep and deal with negative emotions.
- People with poor sleep don't necessarily have more stressors than other people. They react to stressful life circumstances differently and may be more likely to engage in unhealthy coping strategies such as stress-eating.

3

BUSTING SLEEP MYTHS

J ust about everyone has heard about the importance of sleep. It's rampant in the media, but there's a lot of misinformation out there as well. I've encountered many misconceptions about sleep in my practice. Some of them are silly, but many of them can cause unrealistic expectations that lead to disappointment and frustration when they aren't met. Since overachievers are particularly sensitive to not meeting their own or others' standards, and since they tend to be perfectionists, including about their sleep, these myths can contribute to their sleep problems. Here are some of the most common ones along with the science-supported truths.

Sleep Myth #1

I MUST GET EIGHT HOURS OF SLEEP EVERY SINGLE NIGHT TO FEEL REFRESHED, STAY HEALTHY, AND NOT DIE, AT LEAST NOT IN THE NEAR FUTURE.

So many of my patients come in wanting me to help them sleep eight uninterrupted hours every single night. The truth is that eight hours is an average, and just like age-related milestones, or anything else about the human experience that we attach numbers to, there's wide variation. Yet somehow that magic number of eight hours has gone from average to gold standard in our collective consciousness, especially with all of the recent research on the connection between insufficient sleep and dementia.[1]

What is "normal"? The range where most people fall is seven to nine hours, with some people sleeping healthily for as little as six or as much as ten hours per night.[2] I would guess that most of my insomnia patients sleep on the shorter end of that once they finish treatment. Striving to sleep more than their bodies needed before treatment led to them lying awake in bed, which then fed into the insomnia disorder, partially from the body and mind learning not to sleep in bed.

How much sleep should you try to get? Sleep needs vary between individuals and from night to night. If you really wear yourself out during the day, you'll need more sleep. On the other hand, if you have a quiet, relaxing day, you may not need to sleep as much that night. This principle is called the homeostatic sleep drive, homeostatic indicating balance. It's like your hunger drive – if you haven't done it for a while, you want to do more of it.

Look at your own average and how much sleep you need to feel refreshed. That gives you a range to play with, and we'll talk more about how to determine your sleep need below. This is one reason I have people keep sleep diaries: it's enlightening for them to see that how much they've slept during the night doesn't have as much to do with how they feel during the day as they thought it did. If you think keeping a sleep diary will help you figure out your own pattern, go ahead: I've included one for you. If you're concerned that it will draw more attention to your sleep and make you obsess over it, you might not want to keep a diary. And as I mentioned above, don't pay attention to that thing on your wrist – those aren't very accurate and can make people worry more about their sleep.[2]

Sleep Myth #2

A GOOD NIGHT'S SLEEP MEANS NOT WAKING DURING THE NIGHT.

Remember how I said my insomnia patients want me to help them sleep for eight *uninterrupted* hours? You're most likely to do that if you're in your late teens or early twenties. While I do occasionally have patients who are able to sleep without remembering awakenings, it's normal for adults to wake during the night, particularly between sleep stages or sleep cycles.

A few years ago, a book came out summarizing historical research about what sleep looked like before electricity.[3] According to A. Roger Ekirch, people formerly slept in two shifts with a gap of one to three hours in the middle, during which they would engage in social, sexual, or creative activities. Or maybe all three at once. I won't judge.

What did they not do? Freak out, look at the clock, and calculate how much longer they had to sleep before the rooster crowed. Middle-of-the-night awakenings were normal for them. Presumably the pattern has shifted because our sleep is corralled by an abundance of electric light and our 9-to-5 work schedules. I'll talk later about how this isn't everyone's natural schedule, but for now, the takeaway message is if you wake during the night, it may not be a problem, as long as you're able to get back to sleep and feel fine during the day.

Let's talk about "normal" sleep from a physiological perspective. Your brain goes through four stages of sleep during the night, categorized according to whether it's in rapid eye movement (REM) sleep or not.[4] During stage N1, or light transitional sleep, your brain is shutting down for the night. You might notice a sort of floaty feeling. In stage N2, which is where adults spend most of their time, the brain is completely asleep, but not deeply. People with insomnia may still be aware of what's going on around them, which leads to a phenomenon called sleep-state misperception, where someone feels like they're awake, but their brain is actually asleep. It's still sleep, but it's often perceived as not refreshing.

Stage N3, which used to be stages three and four, is what most people think of when they imagine deep sleep. It's known as slow-wave sleep because of the slow, undulating waves on a patient's EEG tracings during this stage. It's very hard to wake someone up from this stage. They're physiologically relaxed as well, with lower blood pressure, lax muscle tone, and slower breathing. This is physically the most restorative sleep stage.

Finally, REM sleep (pronounced as one word, *rem*, not R-E-M, which is a band from Athens, Georgia), is when we have our most vivid dreams. Although our brains are very active in this stage, our muscles are paralyzed, so we don't act out our dreams. REM stands for rapid eye movement, and that's one thing you can look for – are the sleeper's eyes moving beneath their lids? If you've ever watched a baby sleeping, you've perhaps noticed they have a lot of this stage.

When we fall asleep, we cycle through these stages. As the night progresses, slow-wave sleep periods become shorter, and REM periods get longer. That's why you may remember more vivid dreams in the morning and why you may perceive your sleep during the first part of the night as being deeper than in the second half. You're having more slow-wave sleep during the first few hours and more REM sleep during the last few. We typically go through three or four cycles of all the stages, and it's common for adults to wake between these cycles. The hope is that they'll fall back asleep quickly. Hopefully you find it comforting to know that it's normal to wake up during the night and that there's no such thing as a "perfect" night of sleep.

Sleep Myth #3

WE NEED LESS SLEEP AS WE GET OLDER.

While sleep does change as we age, the amount doesn't necessarily shorten. What tends to happen is that we get less slow-wave/stage-three sleep as we age, so sleep quality decreases. When people retire, they lose their external structure, so they may start sleeping later and napping. More daytime sleep leads to less nighttime sleep, which then perpetuates the myth of needing less sleep. I usually recommend that my patients try to keep as regular a sleeping and eating schedule as possible, even after retirement.

Sleep Myth #4

IT'S BEST TO GO TO BED AND GET UP AT THE SAME TIME EVERY DAY.

This myth is half true. One of the physiological systems that controls when we sleep is our circadian rhythm, or our internal clock. It tells us when to be awake, when to be asleep, and when to be hungry. Often, when someone has insomnia, their circadian rhythm gets thrown off, and their body doesn't know what it's supposed to be doing when. The connection between sleep and eating behavior is particularly evident here. I talk to many patients who have little appetite, who don't feel like eating at all in the morning, and/or who find themselves snacking a lot at night. Their bodies have no idea when they're supposed to want food, so they often want it at the "wrong" times – i.e., later in the day, when ideally they'd be eating less – which then perpetuates the problem, because eating is a signal to the body that it's time to be awake. Just like mood, eating and sleep signals go both ways.

The best way to anchor your circadian rhythm isn't bedtime – it's wake time. Sorry, but it's best to wake up at the same time every day. Yes, this can be a challenge, especially for those who have to be up really early for work. Alas, sleeping drastically different schedules on weekdays and weekends can be harmful for your health, as a recent study found.[5]

On the other side, bedtime is more flexible. If you're not sleepy, going to bed when you're "supposed to" leads to you lying awake in bed, which then makes you more likely to develop insomnia because your body and brain are learning that bed is for wake, not sleep. It's best to wait until you're really sleepy and then go to bed, so you'll be more likely to fall asleep quickly.

Remember how I said there's a way to figure out your sleep need? If you keep your wake time consistent, your body will begin to tell you when it wants to go to sleep at night. You can help this process along by giving your body good wake signals – eating and natural light (I'll get to this in a moment) – within an hour of waking.

Sleep Myth #5

YOU KNOW YOU GOT GOOD SLEEP IF YOU DREAMED.

Many of my patients say they don't get good sleep because they don't remember their dreams. Or perhaps they feel they dream too much. However, dreaming is not a good indicator of sleep quality. First, although most of our dreams occur during rapid-eye-movement (REM) sleep, we can dream in any stage. Second, we won't remember our dreams unless we woke during them. That's why some people don't remember any dreams at all. By the way, if you have frequent stress dreams, it is possible to change them through a process called Imagery Rehearsal Therapy, which is really interesting and fun for me as a clinician, but sadly beyond the scope of this book.

Sleep Myth #6

ONLY CHILDREN NEED PRE-BEDTIME ROUTINES.

It's rare in this world of 24/7 stimulation for adults to have set evening routines. If they do, the routines frequently involve some sort of screens, often watching television. It still counts if you watch it on the computer or tablet. Think about when you were a child, or think about your own children if you have them. Small kids have great pre-bedtime routines, usually some variation of bath time, story time, bed, and they're usually sleepier at the end of the routines than they were at the start.

We're no different, we're just bigger. If we do the same sequence of activities before bed every night, our bodies and minds will learn that this routine is a signal that it's time to transition to sleep. Here are some tips for a good pre-bedtime routine:

Eliminate screen use, including television, within one to two hours of bedtime. The light from our electronics is similar in wavelength to sunlight, which is our body's main signal for when it's time to be awake. That's why I recommend getting natural light first thing in the morning if possible. If you must be on a screen late at night for a work emergency, consider using a work-around, like glasses that block blue light, which I'll discuss further below.

One hour before bed, go through your bathroom routine. Maybe that's taking a warm bath or shower, brushing teeth, and putting on pajamas. For the rest of that hour, do something relaxing, but try to do something you only do during that hour and that you can still do if you travel. For example, you might have prayers or meditation you can save for that time, or a certain type of thing you read or listen to only during that period. Just make sure that whatever you're doing, you're not in the bed or bedroom yet.

Again, wait until you're sleepy before you get in the bed.

Once you do go to bed, consider having some sort of mental routine that you implement. I'll discuss some possibilities for what to incorporate in the next chapter.

The hardest recommendation for many people to follow is the elimination of screen use within two hours of bedtime. I'll admit to finding that one challenging, too, especially since it's easy to glance at the phone and get sucked in by one alert or another. There are some work-arounds that may allow you to push screen time to within an hour of bedtime. First, there's a program called F.lux, which you can install on computers and non-Apple tablets and phones, that will turn the screen from blue light to yellow at sunset. It will work on Macintosh computers, but not on iThings. Recent Apple operating systems included a feature called Night Shift, which can be found with the brightness display settings. It does the same thing, and you can set it to start about two hours before your typical bedtime or ten hours before your desired wake time. I recommend you turn the dial to the warmest setting and do the same for F.lux.

As for television, it wouldn't surprise me if manufacturers come up with something similar to F.lux or Night Shift, but for now, the best work-around is glasses that block blue light. You can find them in a range of prices, and none of them are terribly attractive, but they do what they're supposed to, which is to block the blue light signal. They look like yellow or orange safety goggles, and many fit over regular prescription glasses. You'll have to do a little research to figure out which ones are best for you.

By the way, some non-tinted glasses claim to block the blue light signal, but my patients have not found those to be as effective as the ones with colored lenses.

Yes, these work-arounds will help you to push screen time to within an hour of bedtime, but I still strongly recommend going screen-free for that last hour. Why? It's supposed to be a calming time to disengage from the day. It's difficult to allow the mind to wind down when you're still getting emails from work or texts from family or friends, and it's particularly hard not to respond. Even good news can cause emotional arousal. For example, I got news that I'd sold a short story one evening at around 11:45, when I was aiming for bed at midnight. Yes, I broke my own rules and read the email. Yes, I had trouble sleeping because I was excited about the story sale.

Of course everyone is different, and sometimes my patients feel too restricted by the recommendations. Many of my patients have turned their sleep into a full-time job, and they worry about everything from what they should or shouldn't eat or drink in the evenings to what their mattresses and pillows should be. Remember, you don't need to give more than a third of your energy to a process that shouldn't take more than a third of your life (on average).

It takes some trial and error to know which of these rules are the most important for you, and it's okay to be flexible once you know which rules you can fudge and which you can't. Even sleep experts differ on what they will and won't allow. For example, some of my colleagues say it's okay to watch television in bed to help deal with a racing mind. I disagree, but I do tell people they can read in bed for fifteen to twenty minutes to help them make the transition before turning out the light. Don't worry, those aren't the only mind-calming strategies in this book. I'll talk about more as we go along.

Think about trying to find a balance and doing little experiments to see what's important for you. Even if you have to be strict with yourself as you get on track with your sleep, you may not have to be as regimented forever. Good sleep will be the reward for your efforts, and it will motivate you to follow the rules that are most necessary for you.

Of course insomnia is a 24-hour problem, and what

happens during the day affects what goes on at night. You're probably reading this book because you've tried much of what I've recommended – although perhaps not for long enough – and need something more. In the rest of the book, I'll be talking about daytime problems I've helped my overachiever patients with, and which in turn, has helped them to sleep better. In the next chapter, I'll discuss ways for people who have difficulty relaxing to relax. You can incorporate some of the techniques into your pre-bedtime routine, which will help take up some of that last long screen-free hour.

Important Takeaways

- Not everyone needs eight hours of sleep per night.
- It's okay to sleep a little more some nights (like on the weekends).
- It's normal to wake during the night.
- We still need about the same amount of sleep as we get older, though we may sleep more lightly.
- Getting up within an hour of your normal wake time is more important than going to bed at the same time every day.
- Grownups need pre-bedtime routines, too.
- Remembering your dreams tells you nothing about the quality of sleep you got.
- Eliminating screen use for an hour or two before bedtime can help you sleep better.

RELAXATION FOR THOSE WHO CAN'T RELAX

"I can't relax" is a complaint I hear regularly from my insomnia patients. For someone with high achievement drive, the thought of being still and doing nothing can feel stifling and produce panicky feelings. The word *drive* is no accident, because high-achieving individuals often feel like they must be doing something all the time. At a certain point in their lives, that's useful. For example, I knew of several people in graduate school who didn't ever seem to stop. I also knew one who would put Bailey's in their morning cup of coffee.

See? There's a trade-off.

No organism is designed to constantly be in motion or production mode. Even sharks, who are rumored to have to stay swimming in order to be able to keep breathing, have found a way around this.

You may have found yourself eventually crashing and zoning out in front of the television, but not completely allowing yourself to relax, because you feel guilty about taking some time for yourself. Or maybe you allowed yourself to be lost in a book, but rather than enjoying the story, you found your mind wandering to all the things you should be doing. Or, the thing that I most beat myself up about is scrolling through social media at the end of a long day and then feeling bad about the wasted time. Rather than relaxation, I engaged in procrastination. And then I felt worse after.

The problem is not the inability to relax. The problem is that we're using a bad definition and the wrong method.

Thinking about Relaxation in a New Way

The Oxford Dictionary defines relaxation as "The state of being free from tension and anxiety." Wow, this sounds amazing, right? When was the last time you felt free from tension and anxiety?

If you're like me, you may have to think for a minute to come up with a time. The times I can think of when I felt the most relaxed were after massages and facials, or, more recently, after meditation. Don't worry if you just cringed when I mentioned meditation – we'll talk more about that later. Yes, I talk to a lot of people who feel they have "failed" at meditation. Again, the expectations are usually wrong.

So what about that tension and anxiety? We need to dig deeper into the definition, and thankfully, there are more layers. The first sub-definition Oxford gives is "Recreation or rest, especially after a period of work." Okay, that sounds more attainable. It's easier to think about how to engage in recreation or rest, which have simpler connotations, than relaxation. The second sub-definition? "The loss of tension in a part of the body, especially in a muscle when it ceases to contract."[1] That gets down to the basics.

Then there's the second definition of relaxation: "The action of making a rule or restriction less strict."[1] Yes, that applies to very specific situations, but it can still work here. Step back for a moment and look at the "rules" you have for yourself. I'm guessing that a big one, and one that may be driving that feeling of inability to relax, is this:

I MUST BE PRODUCTIVE ALL THE TIME.

Alternately:

FAILURE TO PRODUCE EQUALS FAILURE IN LIFE.

Even if you're not aware of it consciously, do you have that feeling in the center of your chest, like a tightness or force compelling you to do and go and do more and accomplish all the things on your to-do list, which is probably more aspirational than practical? That's one type of psychophysiological arousal, and it can keep you from relaxing, both during your leisure time and when you're trying to sleep.

See what I did there? You say you can't relax, but you do sleep, at least sometimes, even if it's hard. So you must have the ability in there somewhere, even if it takes exhaustion stripping away enough of that arousal for you to get to it. I once remarked to my husband that during stressful periods – and to be honest, they're frequent with my dual career and many recent changes – I seem to have two speeds: either going a million miles a minute and doing everything I have to do . . . or crashing out into sleep.

So how do you – and I – find the middle ground?

Productive Relaxation

Relaxation doesn't necessarily need to be sitting and doing nothing, or even sitting and doing something like reading or watching television. While these activities do have their places – for example, when you're sick or absolutely exhausted and need an escape – it is possible to engage in relaxation but also continue to accomplish things.

Wait, you might be saying, *if I'm accomplishing things, how am I relaxing?* The difference is not necessarily how much you're doing, but what you're doing.

Think about your job or what else you do during the day. If you're an overachiever, it's likely that you're doing well at your job, but it's rare for someone's work to fulfill all of their inner needs and desires. I have encountered a few people, typically academics, who do find great fulfillment in their work and who find it both productive and relaxing. I suspect that's why the emeritus position was created – those individuals just wouldn't retire unless they got to stick around, at least part-time. But for most of us, our day jobs don't give us all the pleasure or fulfillment that we need.

For example, while I enjoy being a psychologist, I'm a strong introvert, so the work wears me out. Don't get me wrong, I'm not shy, as you've probably figured out, and I certainly have no trouble talking to people. But at the end of a long day with patients, I'm ready to go home and not interact with anybody beyond my cat and my husband. If I step back and look at my job, the elements I enjoy most are solving problems, connecting with others, and using my creativity to help people. With that in mind, it's not surprising that I took up writing, first as a relaxation activity and then as a second career. Instead of patients, I have characters with problems that need to be solved in creative and entertaining ways. The marketing side of writing also allows me to use skills that I haven't used since graduate school – skills that I miss, such as testing ads and other experiments to see how I can influence people's buying behavior. Once a researcher, always a researcher, I suppose,

To be honest, sometimes the best part of being an author is that I can manage 90 percent of it from my desk with my cat nearby and not have to interact with anybody face-to-face.

So when you're pondering relaxation activities that might be a little more active, think about what you wish you had more of in your day job and what you wish you could change. Or what you can add. One of the most enjoyable parts of being a psychologist is finding out what people do in their spare time – and how much it differs from their day jobs. For example, you might be a CEO who enjoys reading erotic romance novels for relaxation. Or a professor who does woodworking.

I once had a conversation with someone who was feeling guilty about engaging in a certain activity that was interesting and productive to them – setting up an electronic device for their home – and therefore they didn't feel like they were truly relaxing. I asked them if they felt fulfilled while they were doing it, and they said yes, it was fun. I gave them my blessing to continue. Contrast that with another client of mine who stressed out setting up a new piece of technology. That wasn't relaxing, productive or otherwise.

So, whatever you do for your productive relaxation, rather than feeling guilty about it, embrace it, even if it only makes sense to you.

Relaxation - and Values - Happen in the Present

Another way to approach figuring out a productive relaxation strategy is to ponder your mindfulness values. Uh, oh, did you just cringe when I mentioned the "m" word? Stick with me for a moment. Many people aren't familiar with this aspect of mindfulness, and too often, it gets left out of the pop psychology discussions. Our values can help us bridge the gap between being active and relaxing by helping us figure out what relaxation needs to look like.

Values is a term that gets bandied about a lot, but in this sense, it's the principles you live according to, or "what you want your life to stand for."[2] Our society encourages us to focus more on goals, which can motivate us but can also have the disadvantage of keeping us constantly focused on the future while never feeling good enough in the present. Plus, it can rob us of our joy in accomplishments, which can start to feel anticlimactic. When you're in goal mode, the future-oriented mind is constantly thinking, "What's next?" But relaxation happens in the present. So do values.

One way to determine what your mindfulness values are is to think about goals you're aiming for or have accomplished and the values that drive them. For example, when I was writing my first novel, I was working from the values of creativity and accomplishment. Yes, accomplishment can be a value. When I was interviewing for graduate school, I was warned not to say that helping people was my main motivation for becoming a clinical psychologist, because that's what everybody says. I have a dual bachelor's degree in mathematics and psychology, so it was easy for me to come up with a different answer, namely that I like solving problems, and people problems are the most complex and interesting. So being a psychologist reflects my values of both compassion – since I like helping people – and of problem-solving.

Typically I'll ask my patients to figure out their four core values. They can have more, but the core four are the ones that really drive them. My four are compassion, persistence, creativity, and balance. Admittedly, that last one is aspirational, but that's okay – values don't necessarily need to be principles you're good at enacting, but ones that really resonate with you and that you want to get better at.

Getting back to productive relaxation strategies, your four core values could guide you in choosing what those could be. For example, if you're in a very data-driven job without much human interaction, but you have a value of compassion or connection with others, your productive relaxation strategy could involve some sort of volunteering – for example, coaching a kids' sports team. Or, if you're in a job that involves interacting with people all day, your productive relaxation strategy could be something more solitary, like gardening, cooking, or learning an instrument.

When you are determining what your productive relaxation strategy should be, think about skills that you don't typically practice in your main life. Both of my careers are verbal and cerebral. In other words, I spend a lot of time in my head. One of my favorite relaxing activities is cooking. According to my INFJ Myers-Briggs personality type, extroverted sensing, or awareness of and interaction with what's going on externally, it is my least preferred function. However, doing externally focused and sensory things, like cooking or gardening, bring me into the sensory world, which allows me to use different parts of my brain. And they get me out of my head if I allow them to.

According to some personality theorists, unhealthy coping behaviors come out of the inferior function being activated, so if you engage it in a balanced way, those might be less likely to happen[3]. For example, I'll admit to being a stress eater, which is an unhealthy form of external sensory focus. But if I engage my inferior function in a healthy way, I'm more likely to choose the apple and less likely to go for the cookies. Or neither if I examine whether I'm reaching for a snack out of the desire to self-soothe rather than hunger.

That brings me to the other part of productive relaxation: it involves an outcome that is measurable and detectable. If you're learning a skill, you'll hopefully see yourself improve. If you're making something, or even doing something like coloring, you'll eventually have a finished product, although hopefully you will also give yourself credit for what you're learning along the way. If you're volunteering, the outcome might not be quite so visible, but might instead be appreciation from the people you're helping or a sense of fulfillment.

But what about those days when you're just too exhausted to do anything and need a "real" break? This brings me to my next relaxation strategy.

Intentional Relaxation

I once had an interesting conversation with a patient who was about to start a new semester. This particular person was tempted to label themselves as "lazy" because they enjoy watching television – specifically, binge watching series on their computer. They recognize that they tend to deal with overwhelm through avoidance, which we'll talk about later in the procrastination section, but they also feel guilty when watching television because they are not accomplishing what they feel they should.

As overachievers we tend to keep very hectic schedules. To that end, we need to let go of the idea that relaxation needs to be spontaneous and schedule it instead. As a sleep psychologist, my recommendation is that you schedule relaxation between the second and last hour before bed and then go screen-free the last hour, with a firm pre-bedtime routine.

Scheduling relaxation has a couple of advantages. First, it ensures that you do it. I often find that patients who complain about inability to relax don't allow themselves to do it as a result. That leads to mental crashes, when they engage in activities that they ordinarily would find relaxing but feel guilty about instead. Humans need to relax. We end up with negative health consequences and mental health problems if we don't.

This brings me to the second advantage of intentional relaxation. Rather than crashing as described above, which leads to guilt and more stress, whatever activity you engage in will be relaxing because you're giving yourself permission to do it. I recommend that people mindfully relax, which means that when they are relaxing, they are allowing themselves to keep their minds on what they are doing rather than on the thousand things they feel they still have hanging over them. Yes, this may end up being one more thing to check off the to-do list, but it's an important one.

Physiological Relaxation

Relaxation, like many of the other behaviors we need to engage in for general life satisfaction, is a skill. People tend to beat themselves up over not being able to relax, feeling that something is wrong with them. However, if you think about it, once we get out of the school naptime phase, relaxation is not taught or emphasized. We are a culture that has managed to corral, structure, and put rules on an activity that came more naturally to us as children. So it's time to get back to basics, the ones we engaged in prior to starting school.

If you watch small children breathe, you'll notice that they tend to use their bellies. But at some point, were told to stand or sit up straight, suck in our stomachs, and breathe through our chests. However, chest breathing is stress breathing. What we want to do is learn to breathe through our bellies, which is how we started out.

I have a YouTube video demonstrating diaphragmatic breathing. However, many people end up doing it wrong, because our brains are lazy. This is why dance studios are covered with mirrors. It's not because dancers are vain; rather, when you learn dance, you're making your body move in ways it's not used to, and the brain, rather than learning a new skill, would rather keep up with the old behavior but tell you that you're doing it right, even if you're not. That's why you watch yourself dance in a mirror. All that is to say, it might be helpful for you to watch yourself breathe with a mirror.

Diaphragmatic breathing can be done in any position, so when you're learning, it might be helpful to stand up or lie down, so that you have a bigger range of motion. Put one hand on your chest and one hand on your belly. Ignore any judgmental thoughts you might have about your belly. Watching yourself in the mirror, take a deep breath and then let the breath out. Which hand moved more? Typically when people will do this in my office, the hand on the chest moves more than the hand on the belly.

So what you want to do is first to practice pushing the belly out and then pulling it back in while holding the chest and rib cage still without worrying about your breathing. When you get that muscle motion correct, you can add the breath. Keeping the rib cage still – which means not allowing that top hand to move – inhale and allow the belly to inflate. As you exhale, allow the belly to come back in. Do this for a few breaths, getting used to breathing in what may feel like a completely backwards manner. Then, when you are ready, add a count: Inhale for a slow count of four, then exhale for a slow count of four or more. You'll get a stronger relaxation signal if your exhale is longer than your inhale.

When I'm teaching this at the office, people ask me at this point if they need to pause for a certain count, because they have been practicing – or trying to – different kinds of relaxation breathing. I have not found any benefit to adding a pause to the breath beyond what naturally happens. But honestly, the most important part of this type of breathing is ensuring that you're breathing entirely with the belly and not with the chest.

This is the first in a series of relaxation exercises, and you can build on it easily once you get used to it. My recommendation is that you start doing it for five minutes a day, possibly as part of the pre-bedtime routine. Why five minutes? It's long enough to start getting a response, yet short enough to work into your day. Many of my patients will do it for longer.

Important Takeaways

- You sleep, so your body has the ability to relax.
- Relaxation doesn't necessarily mean sitting still. You can be doing something you enjoy and still relaxing.
- If you need help finding productive relaxation strategies, consider the values, or principles that you live according to. If you're not living according to those values in your everyday work or home life, then engaging in an activity that allows you to act in a value-satisfying way can be relaxing.
- It's not cheating to schedule relaxation. In fact, giving yourself time and space to chill out can help to make it a priority and keep you from falling into traps such as mindlessly scrolling through social media.
- Diaphragmatic breathing is a quick and easy relaxation method.

SLEEP SMARTER – OR, WHAT TO DO ABOUT YOUR RACING MIND

Aside from "I can't sleep," "I can't turn my mind off" is the most common complaint I hear in my practice. But what is mind-racing? Sometimes it's thinking about something stressful, like a meeting you have tomorrow or something that happened during the previous day that you can't let go of. Other times, it's just stuff. You may be planning what to do the next day or obsessing over something that happened in the past. Or maybe you have a song stuck in your head. Whatever it is, it feels like the mind's movement is keeping you from sleeping. So what do you do about it?

One simple strategy to address mind-racing is something we've already talked about. Many of my patients tell me that discontinuing screens within two hours of bedtime helps the brain to feel calmer. There's the blue light, of course, but our screens often have activating – or distressing, if you're a news junkie – content and are associated with attempts at multitasking. That's why it's important to turn off all screens within an hour of bedtime, even if you're using blue light blocking technology.

As much as we may like to think we're not, we are behavioral creatures. Distracting your mind and reading or doing something relaxing before bed – again not on a screen – can also help to calm the brain. This is a great time to do prayers, meditation, or something else calming but still a little engaging. It also trains the brain to think, *hey, now it's time to start transitioning to sleep.*

"I Hate Mindfulness."

One of our most powerful tools for addressing mind-racing is mindfulness. When I talk about mindfulness with my patients, I find that most of them have heard of the concept, and maybe even read a little bit about it, but don't really understand it. Many of them have a misconception that it means having a completely blank mind.

We all know that this is unrealistic. Our minds are busy, and it's impossible to maintain serenity in all instances. Some people also feel that it means being in the moment and only in the moment. Individuals with this incomplete understanding dismiss mindfulness because of what they perceive as a naïve lack of planning. Others feel that mindfulness means not analyzing things, but just accepting them for what they are. We all know that overachievers are very good at analysis, and this ability has helped us to be successful. So why would we want to let go of it? Finally, many of my patients have said that they have tried to meditate, but "they're no good at it." One hallmark of being an overachiever is not liking to fail, so these patients usually give up on meditation before they give it a chance or understand what it's for.

So what are mindfulness and its associated techniques good for? There are already a lot of great books about mindfulness, including on mindfulness and sleep, so I am going to share my favorites techniques and perspectives, and   something that may not be in any other book so far – what my patients have taught me about mindfulness.

The Problem with Why

One of our favorite questions, and one of the queries that drives our racing minds, the stories we tell ourselves, and the stories that get repeated in our culture, is why? Why does somebody behave as they do? Why can't I change this about myself? Why isn't this working like it should? When this question is directed at ourselves, the mind resorts to generalizations, because inaction is easier than action. For example, when we ask, *Why can't I sleep?* the mind tells us that there is some sort of "chemical imbalance" or "something wrong with my brain." When we ask, *Why can't I lose weight?* the answer again comes with a generalization, such as "because I'm lazy." *Why can't I change my approach?* or *Why does this bother me so much?* Because "it's just the way I am."

These generalizations can also happen when we direct "why" questions at others. There is a principle in psychology that says that when we behave in a way we think is bad, we attribute it to the situation. However, when we observe the same behavior in someone else, we often attribute it to something in their character. This may be the only time we are more compassionate with ourselves than with other people. But still, it comes down to a question of *why*.

Wherever you're directing the question, *why* often provokes anxiety. There is something satisfying to figuring out why something is happening – again, it's what our brain likes to do. But often, we come to the wrong interpretation, and then we put too much stock in it.

I would like to propose – and mindfulness encourages us to do this as well – that we ask instead, *Is this useful?* Regarding the past, rather than asking "Why did I do that?" it's more useful to ask, "What can I learn from that?" Regarding the future, rather than asking why something might happen, it's more useful to ask, "What can I plan for or control?" Hint – probably less than we'd like, but the question gives us something concrete to focus on. Finally, when we deal with other people, in most cases, anticipating their thoughts or actions wastes our mental energy because, quite frankly, we're often wrong.

Mindfulness Techniques for the Overachiever

The definition of mindfulness is, rather than just being in the moment, to do so nonjudgmentally, and to focus both internally and externally[1]. Yes, deeming thoughts and behaviors useful or not useful is judgment, but were not assigning a value when we do so. The context matters.

Think about flow experience. When you're in the flow, you're in the moment, you're completely absorbed in what you're doing, and time slips by. That is the most common present-moment focus experience that people can relate to. Think about the last time you were in such a mindset. Were you thinking about the past? Probably not. The future? Perhaps if you were planning something, but if so, it was related to the task at hand, not random worries. Were you fully engaged and focused, able to dismiss distractions? Probably. Mindfulness helps to address the mind racing that often involves the past, the future, and/or judgment by bringing our minds into the present, in a judgment-free mindset.

Tips and Techniques for Bringing Mindfulness into Your Life

My first tip is that mindfulness is a not a technique to help you sleep. In other words, don't try to meditate in bed to put yourself back to sleep. It's often more useful to do it midday, to help you step back from the chaos of your day and therefore to hopefully help you not bring as much of the day's momentum into the evening and into your sleep time. You can use mindfulness techniques before bed, as long as you're not going to end up falling asleep during them. For example, some of my patients like to do just a basic mindful breathing meditation before bed to help them detach from their thoughts.

Tip number 2: Use mindfulness to discover your negative thinking. One mindful principle is diffusion, or decentering, which is when you step back and observe your thoughts. Many of my patients have negative thoughts about sleep: for example, *I wonder if I will sleep tonight*. Of course this is not a useful thought, because the more you focus on sleep, the more you build up anxiety around it.

One of my favorite analogies from Acceptance and Commitment Therapy (ACT) is Tug-of-war with the Monster[2]. In it, one imagines one's thoughts and emotions as a monster standing across a bottomless abyss from you. The monster has one end of the rope, and you're holding the other. You're playing tug-of-war with the monster, because if you can only pull hard enough, the monster will fall into the pit, and then it will leave you alone. The problem is, you're spending a lot of energy and time playing tug-of-war with the monster, but the monster isn't going anywhere. We cannot escape from our thoughts and emotions, so we need to drop the rope. We have to accept that the monster will be there, but we can choose *how* to engage with it.

One part of getting through sleep problems is to realize that, by now, you've likely built up some negative thoughts, emotions, and expectations about sleep. These may occur automatically around bedtime. The thing to remember is that you have a choice about how much you're going to engage with them. Mindfulness can help us to not engage, or to catch ourselves when we have picked up that rope.

Mindfulness tip number 3: Pay attention to the moment with awareness. How many times do you catch yourself not really paying attention to what you're doing? Whether it's coming to a moment of realization when you're driving a familiar route that you haven't really seen anything for the last five minutes, or making a stupid mistake in the kitchen because you haven't been aware of something happening, we tend to slip out of the moment into the past, the future, or a misinterpretation of the present. Awareness, or simply asking *What is happening right now?* can be instrumental into helping us more fully engage with our lives.

Awareness can also help us with our thoughts. One of my patients recently told me that through mindfulness, he's come to realize how repetitive his thoughts are. When he's worried about something, he's noticed that he will go through a thought cycle, not really solve anything, and then go back through those thoughts again. This brings us back to the question, "Are these thoughts useful?"

My next tip is to bring your thoughts back into balance. Sometimes people balk at doing a gratitude exercise, and so I have found one that hits more elements of interest for those of us with an overachiever personality[3]. I can't take credit for it – the reference is at the end of the book – but I found it to be very useful with my patients. It's called the GLAD exercise. The G stands for gratitude, L stands for something you learned, A for something you accomplished, and D for something that delighted you. Once you start practicing the exercise, you may find yourself looking for things to fill in for the next day's GLAD exercise. I found it's definitely more fun to look for things that delight me than things that annoy me.

I have sometimes found that I will talk about mindfulness with my patients during our sessions, and practice and exercise with them, and then at the next session when I ask if they've been practicing at home, they'll say something like, "Yeah, I tried it when I couldn't sleep, and it didn't work." As I mentioned, these techniques are not something to practice to put yourself back to sleep, but they'll also be more useful if you practice them regularly and outside of high-pressure situations. As with learning any new skill, one needs to practice slowly and methodically before calling upon it when you need it. Maybe the first step is to simply notice when your thoughts get the best of you, when you go into those useless and repetitive cycles.

Another way to start with mindfulness is to notice when you're more likely to have trouble sleeping. For example, many of my patients will bring in sleep diaries that show Sunday evening is the worst night. This could be for several reasons. From a physiological perspective, we often disrupt our circadian rhythms on the weekends by sleeping in. It's hard for the body to sleep until 10 o'clock on Sunday morning, and then turn around and go to bed at 10 o'clock on Sunday night. The sleep drive isn't high enough, and the body's internal clock has been thrown off.

From a psychological perspective, many people find themselves dreading the start of the work week. Some of my patients – for example, academics – will start their work week early and try to get a head start on the work on Sunday night. This is often not very good for sleep.

One of my graduate school friends once paid me a very high compliment, which I later came to realize was a sign of me acting mindfully without me realizing it. She told me that when I work, I work hard, and when I play, I play hard. I don't think I was that wild during graduate school, but I was pretty good about shutting off work when I needed to. I had a strict rule (outside of exam or major crunch time) of stopping work by 8 o'clock in the evening. This helped me to manage my stress level.

Do I Need to Start Meditating?

Before we answer the question of whether you need to start a meditation practice, it's important to get on the same page about what meditation is. At its heart, meditation is focusing on just one thing and noticing when the mind is wandering. The point is not to clear the mind, but to notice when the mind wanders and to bring it back. It's not a competition with yourself or anyone else. You may find that on some days, you're able to catch your mind quickly and bring it back. On other days, your mind may be very busy, and it may be several minutes before you bring it back. Either is fine. Again, the important thing is to notice your mind wandering and bring it back – and to practice the noticing and bringing it back. Although I've been meditating for several years now, I still have times when my mind is busier than others.

What if Mindfulness Isn't My Thing?

If you're not connecting with mindfulness, no worries. There are other ways to approach your thoughts.

Sometimes rather than separating from one's thoughts, it can be useful to see what logical fallacies the mind likes to engage in. Some of my patients like this better, and that's fine. When I do cognitive therapy[4], one of the first steps is to identify a patient's thoughts and have them categorize those thoughts as different types of cognitive distortions.

Basically, cognitive distortions are the ways the mind likes to blow up the drama behind certain situations. Our minds are wired for drama. That's why we like fiction, or why we get very caught up with compelling real-life stories. We like to know why people behave as they do, as mentioned above, and we are fascinated by certain people and events. That's why (see what

I'm doing here?) true crime is so fascinating. We want to know *why* criminals do what they do.

There are four main cognitive distortions that I find my overachiever clients tend to engage in. The first one is should statements. This is where you say to yourself, "I should have done this, I shouldn't have done that, I should be more like this." Most of us use should statements to compare ourselves with others, and sometimes we aim should statements at those others. A lot of times when people are doing thought records, they will try to face their thoughts in the form of questions. Questions can be hard to label and work with, so I have them turn those questions into statements. Some of the most popular questions – you can probably guess where this is going – are why questions. Most of the time, why questions can be rephrased into should statements. For example, "Why did I do that?" can be rephrased as, "I should not have done that."

The next most popular cognitive distortion I find with my overachiever clients is all-or-nothing statements. These often reflect an underlying perfectionism, which we'll get to in chapter 6.

Finally, my clients like to engage in a variation of jumping to conclusions, specifically the fortune-teller error, or mind-reading. As the names imply, fortune-teller error entails predicting the future, usually in a negative way, and mind-reading means we assume we know what someone is thinking or feeling.

Often, starting to recognize where our thoughts go in the wrong direction can be useful. The next step is to question our thoughts.

The first question on my list of key questions, or the ones we can ask ourselves to address our illogical thoughts, is "What is the evidence for this thought?" Another one that is particularly good for overachievers is, "Am I holding myself to an unrealistic or unobtainable standard?" Finally, "What are the advantages and disadvantages of thinking this way?" can be helpful for those pesky should statements.

Changing thought patterns is hard. If you need more help, I encourage you to check out a self-help program like Mind over Mood[5] or to seek out your own cognitive-behavioral therapy. Please be aware that many therapists who say they do CBT don't do "real" CBT with homework and thought records.

If you'd like to go further with mindfulness, there are many resources out there. One of my favorites – and one that may be particularly useful for an overachiever – is *The Mindful Way through Anxiety*[6], which is by the authors who wrote the mindfulness treatment manual I use.

However you approach your thoughts, it can be done. As with most things, it takes time and patience.

Important Takeaways

- Instead of asking why questions, ask what questions. For example, instead of asking "Why did I do that?" ask "What can I learn from that?" Also, instead of asking "Why is this happening?" ask, "What can I control about the situation?"
- Don't (just) practice mindfulness at bedtime – practice it throughout the day.
- Use mindfulness to discover your negative thinking – and stop playing tug-of-war with it.
- Pay attention to the moment with awareness.
- Bring your thoughts into balance with a gratitude exercise, such as GLAD.
- The four most popular cognitive distortions that my overachiever patients like to engage in are should statements, all-or-nothing thinking, jumping to conclusions, and mind-reading.

- Three helpful questions to ask of our thoughts include, "What is the evidence for this thought?" "Am I holding myself to an unrealistic or unobtainable standard?" and "What are the advantages and disadvantages of thinking this way?"

PERFECTIONISM

Perfectionism, Part One - I Must Get This Right

I f there was any doubt that I'm a perfectionist, it was erased in the autumn of 2018 after I had surgery. Like a good overachiever, I had prepared my body to guarantee success, or so I thought. I had lost fifteen pounds, I was in the best shape of my adult life, my body fat percentage was lower, my muscle tone was higher, and I was feeling pretty good about myself. The only glitch was I had been under extreme stress trying to decide whether to have the surgery, because my mother-in-law was very ill, so my husband was under a lot of pressure. However, I was experiencing a lot of pain, and something needed to be done, so I decided to have the surgery.

A week after the surgery, a robotic hysterectomy, something went wrong. I was watching television with my husband, and when I lay on my right side, I got short of breath. The feeling went away when I sat up, but I had a distinct sensation of dread. I tried to dismiss it, but I couldn't shake it. I had worked in a pulmonary and critical care practice early in my career, and so I'd heard the horror stories of people dying suddenly from pulmonary embolisms (okay, fine, emboli for you Latin nerds), which are blood clots in the lungs that can cause damage in the lungs or sometimes travel to hearts or brains and cause heart attacks or strokes. It was almost midnight, and no urgent care facilities were open, so off to the emergency room we went. There I found out my blood pressure was higher than I had ever seen it before or since.

Sometimes being a calm mental-health professional isn't the best thing in an emergency room. It meant I had to wait a very long time. But maybe it worked out for the best. When I finally saw a doctor, or he finally saw me, the shift had changed. This particular ER doc decided to order a CT scan, even though he didn't think he would find anything. It revealed a small pulmonary embolism. All right, it was small according to emergency room standards, and I was admitted to the hospital that weekend.

Instead of being grateful that my earlier training had alerted me to the seriousness of the problem I was experiencing, I was annoyed. I had wrecked my perfect recovery, although it was outside my control. I thought I was being active enough to prevent blood clots, but apparently not. Worse, I now had to be on blood thinning medication every day, which was contrary to my self-concept of being a healthy person. Yes, I caught my irrational thoughts, but I still look back on that time with some regret.

A Different Way to Look at Perfectionism

Many overachievers are perfectionists. We like to do things exactly right the very first time we try them. When pressed, we also know how irrational it is. If you ask anyone who identifies as a perfectionist if we truly believe that we must be perfect all the time, we'll probably say no. However, perfectionism does exist, and it gets in our way. For some, it attacks at night with should statements about previous experiences or anxiety about performance the following day.

Please allow me to propose a different definition:

Perfectionism is the bargain we make with ourselves that, if we meet a certain set of conditions, we will be happy.

The dangerous flipside of that is that we make ourselves miserable when we don't meet those conditions. Additionally, we set ourselves up for standards that are impossible to meet.

It's not surprising that we think this way. Many of us grew up practicing some religion or at least are aware of the promise that even if we're not currently happy, we would be in the future. What most people don't realize is that religion challenges us to change our definition of happiness, and it never promises that we will be happy – at least not as we understand happiness in our society.

Taken to its extreme, this attitude of bargaining for happiness results in anxiety and mood disorders. Extreme perfectionism leads to the Faustian bargain of obsessive compulsive disorder, the loss of self to the mental and behavioral rituals that the mind says will guarantee safety, thereby protecting against the dreadful. If you have any doubt of this, read Shala Nicely's book, *Is Fred in the Refrigerator?*[1] She does a beautiful job of illustrating how her perfectionism-driven OCD overtook her life, and then how she moved past it.

When we look back over our lives, we find areas where we failed to be perfect, whether it was getting the perfect job, accomplishing the perfect health recovery, or otherwise meeting some standard or goal that we thought would guarantee happiness. Often these times are opportunities for growth and change, and may have put us on a different path, a better path. I'll talk more about this in my chapter on setbacks. In truth, whenever we do meet those goals or expectations, we don't typically stop to celebrate our accomplishments. The finish line moves, and we are off to the next thing. We rarely allow ourselves to be happy. Yes, happiness is something that we allow ourselves, not something that we earn. We will never ever meet the conditions of this bargain. So what do we do about it?

We procrastinate. Yes, perfectionism is related to procrastination. Just as Voldemort in the Harry Potter series had two faces, so does perfectionism, one of which is procrastination. However, it gets its own chapter.

So let's think about how perfectionism rears its ugly head in our lives.

Perfectionism, Part Two - Imposter Syndrome

Journal entry, April, 2019 –

I went to a new conference last weekend. It was my first time at JordanCon, and my anxiety tried to take over. I had stress dreams, irritability, and a desire to over-prepare. I found myself wanting to read but unable to focus, and I just knew I was going to be found out as the imposter among all those talented people...

Sure, I present as a competent professional, an author, and a psychologist who brings an interesting perspective to any panel conference organizers put me on. But when I look at my book sales – or lack thereof – or the empty spaces on the appointment calendar, I feel far from successful. When somebody calls me accomplished, my immediate inclination is to argue with them. How could I possibly be accomplished? I consistently fall short of my goals, never mind that many of them are outside of my control. I can't make people buy my books. I can't determine whether my patients show up for appointments. I can only control what I do, and theoretically how I react.

The Problem with Comparison

Human beings are hierarchical. If you have any doubt, watch any television show portraying teenagers. They have their categories, their layers of social success, and their varying self-worth. As adults, we still compare ourselves to others to see how we're doing, but we're less obvious about it.

If you're an overachiever, you've probably gotten to the point where comparing yourself isn't helpful, because when you look around, you don't see the people who are trying to achieve the same things you are. As a former therapist pointed out to me, once you get to a certain point, you're striving for goals that very few people have reached. Success owning your own company. Being a best-selling author. Hell, making a decent living being an author is something that is often unattainable, so when you get to a certain point, the only people you see are the ones who made it. We see the successful CEOs, the best-selling authors, the ones who are selling their secrets about how to be successful . . . but it's different for everybody. We don't see the thousands of failures, the masses of people who haven't "made it," whatever that means, or who are still striving. In fact, we often fear being those people.

Perfectionism and Fear of Failure

I read an email from one of those uber-successful authors one weekend when I felt particularly discouraged. In her missive, she said that if you're not as successful as you would like to be, fears stand in your way. I asked my husband, who happened to be standing nearby, what my biggest fear is. Without hesitation, he said "failure."

"Oh, I'm that obvious?"

Again, without skipping a beat: "Yes."

This fear of failure is definitely tied into my imposter

syndrome. Failure, after all, is evidence that I'm not who I present myself to be or who people think I am. Sure, it can be easy to tell someone to look at the evidence, to say, "Count your successes, be grateful for your successes." But the overachiever says, "but look at all that I haven't achieved yet. Look at how far I have to go."

I'm not going to lie: this is exhausting. Running for a finish line that constantly moves further away wears me out. My husband, who as you've probably guessed is an astute observer, once told me he feels like I'm in a race but I don't know who I'm competing against, so I don't know how I'm going to win. I believe at the time I was obsessively checking my book sales, so the answer was probably, "me yesterday" or "other authors in my genre." But there is no winning. There's only surviving to run another day.

So, who are you racing against? And what is your fear? In this chapter, I hope to give you some clues about how you can step out of the race, at least for a little while. Perhaps I'll figure out how to as well. Let's look at some of those perfectionistic bargains that overachievers make with themselves.

Perfectionistic Bargains

BARGAIN NUMBER ONE: IF I FOLLOW THE GURU'S ADVICE, I WILL BE SUCCESSFUL AND HAPPY

It may seem ironic that I'm saying this in a book that is essentially advice on how to sleep better, but when I wrote this section, I was about to see a delayed sleep phase patient – someone whose internal clock is set later than the rest of the world wants it to be – and so the topic was on my mind because so many "gurus" tout rising early as essential for success. Part of being successful is continuing to learn. But it's so easy to get caught in the trap of thinking that implementing the right magical program will guarantee big changes.

There is a lot of advice in the high-achievement/success space about morning routines, specifically the importance of getting up at O-dark-thirty to meditate, exercise, journal . . . you get the idea (and maybe you know the program I'm referring to). The problem is that not everyone's internal clock is set to allow for an hour-long morning routine. When you have to be at work by 8:00, and your body clock is screaming at you that it doesn't want to wake until 9:00, getting up at 5:30 for an extended routine is tough.

I've read those books, and I've gone to those workshops that say the only way succeed as a writer is to get up and write before work. "Your brain will be too tired afterward," they tell us. "Morning writing means that you're prioritizing your writing. Anything that you produce later in the day is crap."

Believe me, I've tried for years to be a "get up early, put butt in chair, and pound out a thousand words before breakfast" writer. My brain clung to the advice that the only way I'd write a bestseller, or at least have a productive writing career, would be to produce words before work. And then what would happen? I'd set my alarm earlier than was reasonable for my circadian rhythm, it would go off in the middle of a dream – which meant I woke groggy and felt crappy – so I went back to bed for another half hour or hour or so. Or my husband would get up and turn off the alarm – the main one is across the bedroom from us, so one of us has to get out of bed to turn it off – and I'd roll over and go back to sleep. Or it would take me too long to drag myself through my supposedly ideal morning routine and I wouldn't have enough time for writing.

Guess what the net result of this strategy was. Hardly any writing aside from some mad scrambles on the weekends, decreased productivity, and feelings of discouragement and frustration. I couldn't follow the advice, and so I couldn't be successful. The fact that I'm a behavioral sleep medicine specialist made me feel even worse. I'm a sleep expert, so I *should* be able to get my schedule under control and force myself into this "ideal" early mold. Well, I couldn't, at least not consistently. It didn't help that my husband is naturally set later, so he will sleep in when he can, and we like to snuggle before getting up in the mornings.

Deadlines are beautiful things, and recently I accepted the idea that if I want to make this next book deadline, I'm going to have to write in the evening even if it's not the ideal time. I have f.lux on my laptop to block most of the blue light, wear blue-light blocking glasses to take care of the rest of it, and write for at least twenty minutes, preferably thirty. Sure, I end up staying up a little later, but then I can sleep until a time my body deems sane. And then I get up and have time for an abbreviated morning routine, sometimes a full one depending on when I need to be at my office or whatever other morning obligation I may have. I'm so much happier now that I'm not fighting my body's preferred schedule, and I'm finding it easier to get up at a more consistent time on weekends, too, since I'm not feeling as sleep deprived.

And guess what? The words I write after dinner are not crap. In fact, this creative time is part of my winding down routine, and I go to bed happier because I've done something meaningful and fulfilling.

I understand that not everyone can sleep on their ideal schedule. Whenever I do talks about circadian rhythm disorders, I poll the audience. First I ask how many of them have a natural sleep schedule that meets our culture's "ideal" of going to bed at 10:00 and waking up at 6:00. About a third to a half of the audience raises their hands. Then I ask how many of them would still have that schedule if it hadn't been beaten into them by their children's school demands. About half of the original responders say yes again. That means only a quarter to a sixth of the audience are naturally early birds. The rest of us have internal clocks that are set slightly or a lot later.

So what do you do if you have to keep an earlier schedule than your body prefers? Adjust life as much as possible and stop stressing about the rules that aren't useful to you. If you don't have trouble sleeping, then sleeping in on the weekends may not be so bad. There was a study out of Sweden[2] demonstrating that, for people who are chronically sleep-deprived during the week, sleeping a little later on the weekends can be helpful. Michael Breus in his book on chronotypes[3] recommends no more than an hour's variation in wake time, but at least it's something.

This is good advice to follow about most other advice – keep what's useful and don't stress about the rest. Yes, it's hard not to fall into that perfectionism and the seduction of the "if you only do X, you'll be successful" formula. Whether or not your morning is miraculous, the important thing is for you to get the sleep you need and accomplish what's meaningful to you, regardless of when you do it.

BARGAIN NUMBER TWO: IF I KNOW WHAT TO EXPECT, I'LL BE CALMER AND MORE IN CONTROL OF THE OUTCOME

I admit to being one of those authors who checks my books' sales numbers and rankings obsessively. When I'm selling books, I feel good about myself. When I'm not, I don't. Book sales have factored into the bargain I've made with myself that if I can only sell enough books to make a side income, I can be happy. One of the problems with our brains is that uncertainty is less tolerable than unhappiness. Consequently, if we are unsure whether we will succeed at something, we often set ourselves up for failure. We may not have gotten what we wanted, but at least we could anticipate the outcome. This is self-sabotage.

For the risk-averse overachiever, this can be deadly and result in stalled careers or worse. As we progress in our lives, the risks get bigger and the prizes get better. But we fear failing at them.

Here's my personal example. When I first got published, I had the same dreams that many first-time authors have: I would "catch lightning in a bottle," as someone put it, and my book would magically be a bestseller and optioned for a movie. I would be able to quit my day job and write full time. Of course that didn't happen. Nor did it happen with my second, third, fifth, or even tenth book. I've now published sixteen novella- and novel-length works of fiction and one full-length nonfiction book, and I still rely on my day job.

I do have hopes for this overachiever book, but that has worked against me. I have been working on this book for over two years, probably longer. What has gotten in my way? Definitely procrastination, but also self-sabotage, or getting in my own way. One could argue that they are the same thing, but I'll get more into procrastination later, which entails a certain type of self-sabotage. This delay has come from the second perfectionistic bargain — if I don't write the book (self-sabotage), I'll know what to expect (nothing), and therefore I won't have to fear failure.

Self-sabotage becomes even more of a problem when you've experienced major disappointment in the past. In summer and autumn of 2018, I released the *Dream Weavers & Truth Seekers* urban fantasy series under my pen name, Cecilia Dominic. I thought this series would be THE ONE, my big break. I spent a lot of money on beautiful covers, hired a publicity company to help me with releases, and did what I thought were all the right things. I made some mistakes, most notably releasing the first two books of the series during the summer, which is always a slow time for book sales. I also hit some bad luck. I had the misfortune of releasing the books when Amazon was making a lot of changes, which negatively impacted author sales almost across the board. I'm pretty sure the problem isn't the books themselves. The people who read them loved them, and the reviews are good. The third book, *Web of Truth*, was a finalist in the prestigious Daphne du Maurier writing contest, which shows that it's good. But sales were, well . . . .

Yeah, the series flopped. I didn't realize just how much this affected me until I went to start on my next project and was paralyzed. I developed the self-sabotaging thought, "nobody really cares what I have to say." This has, of course, made writing very difficult, although as I push through and write more, it gets better. Thankfully, my mindfulness practice has allowed me the ability to observe my thoughts, and, when I get in my own way, I can catch myself and try not to choose certainty over progress. I also remind myself of what I now know that I didn't know before.

That's one thing I know I can expect from every book release or any other risk I take – I will learn something important, and I can do what I need to do to make it better next time. But wow, it's hard to get past that uncertainty. Again, I have to remind myself that the point is to create, and I need to focus on what I can control.

How does self-sabotage affect sleep? I've had patients who were so disappointed by repeated "failures" to have the perfect night that they worked against themselves and intentionally didn't follow treatment recommendations correctly. They may not have been sleeping well, but at least they knew what to expect.

BARGAIN NUMBER THREE: IF EXPECTATIONS ARE TOO HIGH, I WILL DISAPPOINT.

Or: *If I always meet or exceed expectations, I will feel secure.*

At the beginning of the chapter, I mentioned the race that we are all running against ourselves. This could also be considered part of the bargain: that if we could only meet a certain set of conditions, we can be happy. We continually focus on how far we have to go, not on how far we have come. I have seen this with many patients who have recovered from serious head injuries. They tend to be very frustrated about their limitations and struggles, and when I call their attention to how far they have come, they feel better.

Many times, overachievers feel uncomfortable when others admire or compliment them. I cringe when anybody uses the term *accomplished* to describe me. I certainly don't feel accomplished, mostly because I ignore what I have achieved in favor of what I still want to.

Several of my overachieving patients have expressed a similar discomfort with compliments. When we dig deeper, many times it comes out that they're afraid of disappointing whoever the other person is. Perhaps they fear that high expectations set them up for a greater chance of failure. This brings us to another aspect of that bargain, which is that I must not disappoint or fall short of what other people expect of me. Another way of looking at it is that, for some people, they must always win, which will of course guarantee that others respect them (but probably not).

Some of my patients engage in excessive reassurance seeking, which fits in with the overachiever's need for feedback and approval. Often this comes in the form of repeating the phrase, "you know?" several times in conversation. I've noticed this in session. Sometimes I have kept count of how many times a client has inserted that question into their speech, and I'll tell them every ten or so *you know?*'s. Many times they are shocked, and then they start catching themselves. Yes, we desire to be understood, but it can get excessive.

Reassurance-seeking and desiring complements both have the same problem at their hearts, which is that we allow others too much power over how we see ourselves. Achievements can only happen in context, right? And we also know that we believe things that come from others more than we believe what we generate ourselves. Consequently, we can fall into the trap of allowing others to determine what makes us perfect. And just as with seeing good book sales, getting reassurance provides that little hit of dopamine that keeps us addicted to it.

Rather than allowing others to determine whether we are or are not perfect, perhaps a better question is to see whether we can allow ourselves to be simply good enough. The over-achiever tendency toward guilt can make this tough. Good enough is never enough, but perfect is impossible, so what do you do?

Here's a scary idea – practice being imperfect. You may have just laughed and said or thought, "I practice that all the time, because I'm never perfect." Allow me to clarify: *deliberately* practice being imperfect. When my clients have done this, they've found it to be freeing. It could be something simple and mostly hidden, like wearing mismatched socks. Or it could be something more obvious, like leaving the house without makeup on or with mismatched earrings. You could also catch yourself when behavior tips from cautious to fearfully obses-sive. For example, many clients have told me that they take too long to send emails because they check them over several times. While you may not want to intentionally send out emails with typos, perhaps you could check them only once or twice.

Emails and texts give us opportunities to practice imperfec-tion without planning for it. For example, at one point last year, I dictated an email to my fiction newsletter list, and although I read through it and thought I cleaned it up, the newsletter went out with a somewhat scrambled sentence in the worst place: a book description. When I got the newsletter – they all come to me when they go out to my list – I saw the mistake, and my heart sank. What would they think of me? Of my book? My first impulse was to send out a correction, but instead, I recognized the opportunity to practice imperfection and decided to wait and see if anyone said anything. No one did. I engaged in mindful self-compassion and nonjudgmental observation, and I did not say anything about it until the following week's newsletter. I apologized for the typo, and I may have said something about deciding to practice imperfection.

So, how can you practice imperfection today?

BARGAIN NUMBER FOUR: IF I SUCCEED ON THE FIRST TRY, IT MEANS I'M A SUCCESSFUL _____

Flip side: if I don't succeed right away, I'm destined to fail.

The beginning of Daylight Savings Time in the spring is always a tough time for my patients. One year I got an especially clear picture of just how much, because I was on vacation for the week immediately after the shift. No, I didn't plan that intentionally, but it worked out nicely. My colleague covered for me while I was out, but she didn't get any calls, surprisingly. When I returned to work on March 18, I had the benefit of looking at sleep diaries from the week(s) before DST started and from the week after at the same time. Pretty much everyone had trouble, and the contrast couldn't have been clearer. I ended up having the following conversation with almost everyone:

"So it looks like you were going along really well before the time change."

"Yes, and I'm so frustrated!"

"Because . . . ?"

"I was doing so well, like you said. And then the clocks shifted, and my sleep got messed up again. I feel like I'm back to square one."

"Well, I would call it square one and a half, so don't be discouraged. It's pretty much you and everyone else."

(With relief) "Really? Other people are having this trouble?"

"Yes, I've had this conversation with almost everyone else this week."

"Oh, that makes me feel so much better. And you're right, I need to do better about . . . ."

ONE PATIENT SURPRISED ME. She'd had a few rough nights after DST started, coupled with trying to decrease her sleep medication. But instead of expressing discouragement, she started by saying, "You'll be proud of me."

"How so?" I asked, intrigued.

"Well, instead of beating myself up, I told myself it was a temporary setback, and I can try this again. I haven't completely failed."

She was right, and it helped me to recognize another lie that overachievers tell themselves, a fallacy that's driven by the need to accomplish whatever task we're facing at all costs: that we have just one shot to get something right or to accomplish something. Perhaps it's partially because in so many movies, the climax comes down to getting something right at the crucial moment. Winning the big fight or game. Completing the big project. The grand romantic gesture.

But in our lives, how many times do we only have one shot to get things right? Sure, there are certain circumstances, but those are rare, or at least, not everyday occurrences – pulling the jump cord on the chute, nailing the big presentation for a prospective client, making the big argument in court. Of the three examples I just gave, the only one that's life or death is the parachute one. One of my dietitian colleagues mentioned that she's seeing a former client of mine, who said the main thing she remembered from her work with me was me asking, "What's the worst thing that could happen? Are you going to die?" She told the dietitian she's found a lot of comfort in that statement.

As I mentioned in the last section, while we may not get to do specific situations over, we can at least learn from them for the next time.

I've struggled with this fallacy in several areas of my life. In an article I refer to in my procrastination talk and chapter[4], the author argues that writers are often people for whom success has come easily. And growing up, that was the case. As one of my friends joked, "A is for Anne Always." Of course it wasn't, but that's how it looked, and I liked that reputation and the feeling that came with it.

As I mentioned in a previous section, the book series I released in 2018 flopped, and so did my confidence. I felt as if I'd failed at my shot at writing success, so there was no point in continuing to try; I went into a season of paralyzing self-doubt. It was a valuable lesson to me that I'm subject to many of the fallacies I work on with others, and even though my reaction could be considered a mistake, I learned something valuable about myself. I also rediscovered the joy in the creative process of my writing, which is the most important part.

PERFECTIONISM CAN START to become an identity if we're not careful. By practicing imperfection and embracing failures – more about that in the setback chapter – we can learn to be gentler with ourselves. Perhaps we can see the opposite of perfectionism as a type of self-compassion. We are all works in progress, and if you think about it, that's okay. Overachievers like a challenge, and it's fine and admirable to want to improve oneself. As in all things, balance is key.

Important Takeaways

- We can think of perfectionism as the bargains we make with ourselves to try and guarantee happiness.
- Even if someone is an expert, their advice isn't for everyone.
- There is no way to know or control what will happen.
- It is impossible to meet everyone's expectations, especially our own.
- If you don't succeed on the first try, you can still be successful.
- Practice being imperfect. It's easier than being perfect and gives us opportunities to grow.

TIME MANAGEMENT

The Tyranny of Time

I remember the moment in my life when I felt like I had more things to do than I had time for. I was in my early forties, my practice was booming, the demands of my writing career were increasing, and suddenly I was dealing with my own health issues and a sick mother-in-law. The to-do list loomed large, and it felt like I was living in a giant game of whack-a-mole.

I'm surprised it took so long for this to happen – maybe because I don't have the responsibility of children on top of everything else. Still, when it comes to the expression, "If you want something done, give it to a busy person," I and many overachievers are the ones others think of. Why wouldn't you give us more work? Theoretically, we can do it well and in a timely manner, maybe even beyond what you're hoping for or expecting, no matter how much other stuff we have going on. The problem? There's always a price.

One of the ways overachievers pay is the to-do list that likes to pounce on you once you're about to drift to sleep.

Step One: Acknowledging What We Do

When I sat down to put together a talk on self-care – one of the many things on my to-do list, but one with a deadline, so it was getting done first – I wrote out my roles as an example. And I kept writing. And writing. And writing some more. Being a psychologist, entrepreneur, author, speaker, wife, cat-mom. . . . Well, you get the picture. Here's part of my list, from the practice:

Full-Time clinical provider
Administrative supervisor
HR department
IT department
Inventory manager
Clinical director
Equipment manager
Compliance officer
Marketing director
Sales analyst
Speaker
Author

And that's just at work. In most companies, a different person or department handles each role. When you work for yourself, you're everything, at least at first. I do have an office manager – thank goodness – but there's still much to be done. I have another list for home, although thankfully that gets split with my husband.

You may not have my exact situation, but I'm guessing you, too, feel overwhelmed by your to-do list, which can end up being a "should have been done yesterday" list. In this chapter, I'm going to share some of the time management and prioritization tools I use myself, the same tools that have helped my clients to bring the list under control –or at least to keep it from controlling them. But first, let's discuss some of the traps I have observed my patients falling into. I'll admit, I get snared by them, too.

Time Trap #1: I Have to Clear the Deck

I once had a patient who would come in week after week and complain, "I never get anything done." When we explored this further, we found that she was getting things done – just not what she wanted to accomplish.

"You sound like you're very productive," I observed. "What's making you feel constantly behind?"

"Well, I have these big projects I have to do," she said. "And I prioritize them, but I don't ever get to them."

I asked what she meant by prioritize, and she said, "Well, I try to get all the other stuff out of the way first, but then more stuff comes up, and when I'm finally finished, it's time to go home."

It makes sense to want to "clear the deck" in order to focus, but the truth is, the deck will never be clear. So how do you manage all those little tasks and deal with the ones that come up?

First, learn to recognize what's important, what's urgent, and what's an emergency. If you'll recall from the first chapter, overachievers often have trouble differentiating between what's important and what's urgent. I didn't really grasp the difference between the two myself until I read Steven Covey's book *The 7 Habits of Highly Effective People*[1]. Urgent tasks, he explains, are those with time limitations on them. That voicemail message from a patient or client, for example, might be an urgent task. Obviously those can't be ignored for too long. Important tasks are the ones that reflect your values (remember those from the relaxation chapter?) and help you achieve your long-term goals.

They're the big projects that help to move your life and work forward in a meaningful direction. Emergencies usually make themselves clear, but just in case: emergencies are those things you can't ignore without putting your health or safety at risk – or the health or safety of others.

Second, get what you can out of the way. I really like what David Allen advises in his book *Getting Things Done: The Art of Stress-Free Productivity*[2]. He advises sorting tasks between those that can be accomplished in under two minutes and those that will take longer. The tiny tasks? Do them right away. The bigger tasks? Schedule time for them.

Sometimes it can be helpful to touch the big projects, which will get you in the right frame of mind to work on them in the middle of the smaller stuff. I had an example of the value of this strategy one afternoon recently. I had about an hour and a half between two phone meetings, and I had several tasks on my list, including sending a W-9 to a book vendor. This required me to fill out a new form with an account number I had to look up, enter the day's charges and payments into Quickbooks, give the financial sheet to my office manager so she could bill insurance, prepare for my second call. . . . Oh, and I also needed to buckle down and work on this book, since it was due to my editor within a week. I chose to deal with the small things during that time, because I knew I'd have time after the calls, but I did something that would increase the likelihood that I would, indeed, write rather than packing up and heading home for the day.

I started writing this section before my second phone call. That way, I got the activity into my brain, and it felt like it was waiting for me, which turned it into an urgent task rather than just an important one. I touched it and kept it to a small thing – just one section. Now that I've finished this one small but important task, I can move on to my after-work errands feeling like I've accomplished something. Perhaps I'll get a cookie. I'll also be more likely to get back to the chapter during my designated writing time this evening, because the ideas are flowing.

Time Trap #2: The Myth of Uninterrupted Hours

If I only had a few uninterrupted hours....

How many times have we said that? Or thought it? I know I used to think that way, especially before I became a published author. It felt like the only way to be productive, especially when it came to big projects, was to have several hours back-to-back when I could work without being disturbed. And it's true, I was able to work like that sometimes, but how often does life allow us long stretches of uninterrupted time?

I used to do an exercise with my clients who felt they were wasting time. It involved them keeping track of how they were spending their hours, in 15-minute increments. The ones who managed to follow the instructions found they had – and wasted – more time than they realized. This was in the days before smartphones, social media, and other time-sucking devices and activities, so I can only imagine what this exercise would look like now. I stopped making this assignment, because it was too labor intensive for my clients, but it's something I challenged myself to do recently. I didn't even make it for a day. It's difficult to step back and see how we're truly using our time.

There's nothing like a deadline to make you find time you didn't know you had. When I got the contract for my third fiction book, *Blood's Shadow*, I found myself in a busy period at the practice, and I would often be exhausted when I got home. I'm sure I did have some long stretches of time, but my recollection of writing that book is doing so in twenty- to thirty-minute increments before leaving for work. Bestselling fiction and nonfiction author Joanna Penn calls this "writing in the margins." I called it "writing in the corners" before I read her term[3], but it all means the same: using small slices of time when you're not doing anything else and might otherwise be wasting time.

I would also like to point out that that strategy worked at that particular time in my life. It doesn't anymore. It's okay to change systems and strategies depending on life demands.

So rather than attempting to carve out large chunks of time to accomplish something, try breaking it down into small enough pieces to do in the margins or corners of your day. You may be surprised by the time you find.

Time Trap #3: Failure to Plan

When I was doing Weight Watchers before my wedding, one group leader in particular kept saying, "Failure to plan is planning to fail." I later tried to find the origin of that quote for my *Business Basics for Private Practice* book[4] and couldn't, but the sentiment is true. When we go into our days without a plan, it's no wonder we get caught up in the urgent and not-so-urgent, then miss out on opportunities to accomplish the important things.

I recently had a conversation with a patient who was complaining about not working as efficiently as they used to. When I asked where they felt they were slowed down, they said that the nature of their job is such that they have stretches of time when they're waiting for something to finish, and so they'll do something else. Then they forget to check on the first thing, which means it goes longer than it should, and sometimes they have to repeat it. This reminded me of a certain scenario at my house – and the reason I don't do laundry anymore: I would put a load in the washing machine, start writing, get distracted by something else or several somethings, and forget about the clothes in the washing machine, sometimes for days. That was in the days before we carried around devices with reminders, but, to this day, my husband still does the laundry. I'm okay with this. For my patient, however, I suggested they use a timer.

I also asked this client whether they set out their agenda at the start of the day. Did they know what they wanted or needed to accomplish? The answer was no.

Have you ever experienced the phenomenon of knowing you have a lot to do, but then coming upon an unexpected bit of free time and freezing because you can't recall any of the things on your must-do list? Or looked at the sheer number of tasks and not known which to do first? Or do you have so many lists they've ceased to be useful?

Let's talk about agenda-setting, but in a different way than what you've probably heard before.

Time Prioritization

When we look at our to-do lists, they can seem overwhelming. You may step back and think, "Oh, crap, how am I going to get all this done?" Again, one of the difficulties overachievers tend to have is distinguishing between what's important and what's urgent. But we need to do both, and if we don't, we end up dealing with evening- and weekend-eating monsters when we'd benefit more from relaxing.

There have been many time-management prioritization techniques proposed over the past several decades. Two of the big ones are Alan Lakein's ABC list[5], which I originally learned in graduate school, and Steven Covey's four-quadrant categorization. I like both of these, but I've found that adding another layer to these models can help bring things under control.

So what do we do?

First, we figure out what the monsters are. Do you have big projects looming? Something you've been needing to do that keeps getting pushed down the list? Some little things that keep bugging you, but that you can't seem to remember when you have a few spare minutes to do them? Let's make a list – but before you start writing stuff down, take a sheet of paper and fold it in half vertically, so there's a line running down the middle, from top to bottom. Now dump everything you have to do on the left-hand side of the paper. Go ahead. I'll wait.

GOT YOUR LIST? Good. Now, on the right side of the paper, write the first step you need to take toward addressing or accomplishing the item on the left-hand side. Not all the steps, just the first one. You can't do the second step until you do the first one, so don't waste your mental energy.

This is a technique, straight from the insomnia treatment world, called the Worry Log[6]. It helps the mind to focus on more immediate tasks rather than spinning through large problems.

Okay, now it's time to prioritize. You're going to label each of the items on the right-hand side – the first steps – according to the following:

A) absolutely must be done today
B) before the end of tomorrow
C) can wait. . . .

Look familiar? Yep, that's the Lakein ABC prioritization scheme[5], but I add another letter: D for delegate.

Another issue many overachievers have is trouble delegating. I suspect that's because we don't want to have to go through the trouble or hassle of training someone to do something. But think about the time and effort you could save yourself if you did delegate. It may be something like hiring someone to clean your house or to fix that squeaky floorboard. Or maybe paying for one of those prepared food services so you don't have to worry about cooking as much, or so you don't eat out as often. At work, you could give more tasks to an assistant or administrator. For example, I now have my office manager do the reference lists for most of my talks, since it's time-consuming, and my time could be better spent. Maybe you could hire a bookkeeper for your small business, so you don't have to enter every single receipt, and they can alert you to things you may be missing.

Now that you know the prioritization scheme, there are a couple of restrictions. You can only have three A tasks, unless they'll take less than 5 minutes apiece, in which case you can have five. If you finish your A's, you can go on to your B's, which you can only have three to five of, as per the previous rules. Write out your A tasks on one sheet of paper and put the others away in a planner or somewhere else you can find them. There's your three-to-five-item single-step to-do list. Isn't that more manageable than that list of ten, twenty, fifty things?

I typically encourage my patients to do their agenda-setting the day before or the morning of the day that the A tasks will be accomplished. That way you won't end up sitting there thinking, "Now what was I supposed to do?"

As for those big tasks, where do you put them? Steven Covey recommends plotting out your schedule by week, and I've found this to be useful as well. I also have monthly goals that I set. That way if I do find myself in that "what to do?" mode, perhaps if I've finished my A and B tasks, I can look at my monthly or weekly agenda and figure out what needs to happen next. The monthly or weekly agenda can also be a good place for those things you put on the left side of the paper.

Finally, some people have found time-blocking to be useful, although many of my overachiever patients find it tough to stop doing tasks when the end of the block of time arrives.

You may find that some time management advice is useful and some isn't, so I encourage you to experiment and see what works best for you. If you're doing what you need to do, it doesn't matter if it has a letter attached to it or some other method. Who knows? You may come up with the next big development in time-managing strategy.

Going back to the chapter on relaxation, one thing to keep in mind is to plan self-care time. All the time management in the world won't help if you're burning yourself out.

Say No to Burnout

When I was putting together a talk on burnout and compassion fatigue in dentists, I came across an interesting finding. In some countries, the likelihood of burnout is lower for older dentists than for younger ones. This is interesting, because one would assume that the longer you've been in a field, the more likely you are to experience burnout. The authors didn't speculate about why the opposite was true for this particular group, but I have a theory: The older we get, the more likely we are to learn how to say no.

In the past year or so, since having children has been off the table, I've been pondering what I want my life to look like. To that end, I've stepped back and reassessed, and I feel like I've gotten a much clearer idea of what I am and am not willing to do. Now when I'm faced with a new obligation or big decision, my first question is, "Will this contribute to my long-term goals?"

How did I decide on my long-term goals? I look to those who are living what I consider the dream life, and I figure out how that picture aligns with my values. For example, I follow the Creative Penn podcast, and Joanna Penn's primary value is freedom. She writes books, hosts her podcasts, and does a lot of traveling. As someone who's tied to an office all day and who would like the ability to, as she says, "read, write and travel when I want," I resonate with her value. It sounds amazing.

My other core values are integrity, compassion, creativity, learning, persistence, and balance. If I'm feeling that core sense of exhaustion, it typically means I'm violating one or more of those values – typically balance. That one's more aspirational than practiced, and I catch myself falling into the traps I mentioned in the relaxation chapter. I've even uninstalled Instagram from my phone when book deadlines approach, since I can spend hours scrolling through its mostly politics-free collection of kitten pictures and videos, amazing food and wine pictures, and photographs of amazing places. As someone reminded me recently, that's "empty" relaxation time, when I'm not fulfilling any values, and I end up feeling worse afterward. Sure, it may be fun to peek in on others' lives, but not if their lives make me feel badly about my own.

What does it look like to make choices that align with values, in the name of helping life progress and not burning out, in everyday life? Sometimes it's not so obvious. Here's an example. I was recently recruited to join an executive coaching team. It's an exciting opportunity, but before I committed, I had to ask myself, "Will this contribute to my long-term goal of increasing revenue outside of direct client hours?" At first the answer seemed to be no. I'd be signing on for more client hours, not less. But then I had to consider the contacts and opportunities being on this team would give me. I'd be meeting executives from large companies, who may then invite me to give talks and workshops. Those make more money with less face-to-face time, so I said yes.

ONE THING I would like to caution you against is the trap of deeming yourself disciplined or not disciplined enough to engage in time management methods. As I'll discuss in the procrastination chapter, willpower or discipline is not a finite resource, although our minds tell us it is. Instead, focus on developing routines. Once something becomes a routine or habit, it takes less effort and feels easier.

There are many time management books, strategies, and pieces of advice in the world. We're all unique, and we each resonate with different things. A strategy that makes sense for me may not do so for you, and vice versa. This is one area where it's easy to fall into a variant of one of the traps I discussed in the previous chapter: that if something doesn't work right away, I must not be good at it. Be patient with yourself, give yourself time, explore, and experiment. Remember, time management is likely not a life-or-death thing, although the mind may treat it that way. You may also need to change your strategies as you grow and your life circumstances evolve, and that's okay. That's one of the advantages of being human.

Important Takeaways

Avoid these productivity pitfalls:

- Trying to clearing the decks before starting.
- Waiting for large swathes of uninterrupted time.
- Not "using the margins."
- Not making a plan.
- Not saying no enough.
- Deeming yourself undisciplined when what you really need is routines.

HANDLING THE INEVITABLE – FAILURE AND SETBACKS

There's a joke that regularly comes up on the internet about how the brain likes to bring up mistakes from several years ago right as we're trying to fall asleep or go back to sleep. It's a funny and popular joke because this is such a common human experience. The problem is that the experience of failure is also unavoidable no matter how good, proficient, or – dare I say – expert we become.

For example, my husband and I enjoy attending concerts given by the Atlanta Symphony Orchestra. In 2019, we attended one that featured the principal oboist Elizabeth Koch Tisione in an oboe concerto. Yes, there are oboe concertos. She came out, stood at the music stand, and the orchestra began to play. Her part came in, and then something strange happened. The sheet music in front of her kept turning back. The stage person had set the music stand in a draught.

Koch Tisione kept trying to play, but after fighting the music for a few minutes, she and the conductor came to a mutual agreement to stop the piece. She calmly moved the music stand, and they picked up again. The music was gorgeous, and as far as I can tell, she played flawlessly in spite of what some may term as a setback. She got a standing ovation, and the conductor made a show of throwing the music on the ground.

Ms. Koch Tisione is a professional, and as such, has learned to pick right back up after course-correcting from a setback. She had no control over where the music was placed. Or perhaps she did, and the airflow in Symphony Hall was strange that night. Whatever the reason, things didn't go quite as planned, but she didn't let it fluster her. I suspect that she became the favorite Atlanta Symphony Orchestra musician of many in the audience that evening.

One of the phrases I hear repeatedly in my office is, "It wasn't supposed to be this way." Whether it's a professional setback or a personal one, it's hard when life throws us off our path, especially for the overachiever who likes to know what's ahead and is poised for accomplishment and success. But setbacks are inevitable. The question is how we handle them.

Step Out of the Script

If you were to step outside of your life and look at it as a whole, what would you see beyond where you are now? Are you pretty sure you know what will happen? Or what you want to happen?

There's a song by the Godfathers called "Birth, School, Work, Death." That seems to be a pretty good summary or bullet point outline, but beyond that, we don't really know, and it's less under our control than we'd like to believe. Overachievers have an interesting quandary in that they like to know what's coming, but they also need to be challenged to stay interested.

Having kids has always been part of my script. Thanks to biological limitations, that didn't happen, and I've been dealing for the past five years with my script getting changed. As I alluded to previously, it all culminated with a hysterectomy – or as I called it, a uterine eviction – in September 2018. Obviously that removed any chance of us having children without prior planning and lots of extra effort, so I've been working on redefining what I want my life to look like as I continue through my forties and beyond.

I will admit, I did not handle my script change well. The problem was that I wasn't just dealing with my script. The issue came from the fact that it's society's script for women, and it's hard to find a different one. Remember, I'm an overachiever, and I like approval. I grew up in a traditional family and a traditional neighborhood in the 1980's. The women around us worked, but they also parented. I got the clear message that woman are expected to do it all and be good at it. When my body couldn't even manage to make a baby, I felt as if I had not only failed, but I was flawed in some way. The word *defective* floated through my mind on more than one occasion. It was not a good feeling.

This script, or shall we even say prescription, to have children is powerful. During the time I struggled most with my infertility, I wrote and published several fiction books and one nonfiction book, continued to grow my practice and my reputation as a clinician and speaker, and overall had what many would consider to be a successful life. But I felt like an imposter.

I finally sought therapy, and after a couple of false starts, found a woman I could work with who understood. I still mourn the fact that I never had children – and that my inability to have children feels like a failure to achieve something important – but I no longer feel defective.

My point in telling this story is to show that no matter how successful someone seems, they're probably dealing with something strong and negative in some area. I also want to encourage you, if you're struggling, to seek the help you need, even if it takes a few tries.

Plan, but Don't Worry – Setbacks Can Be Opportunities in Disguise

One of my patients who is entering his sixth decade said something interesting to me recently. He noted that when he was in his thirties, he was very focused on making sure he had the next step in his career lined up so he could continue on his track toward advancement. Now that he's older, he trusts that the next opportunity will come along when it's time, and so he's less focused on what happens next.

Yes, it's necessary to plan for the future. But how much time do we waste worrying about it?

I can appreciate this perspective. When I was in graduate school, I planned to go into academia as an alcohol researcher – studying it, not drinking it, although I'll admit that happened, too. But during my third year, I failed to match for internship the first time I tried. This was a giant setback, or at least it felt like it at the time. The rest of my cohort went away to internship, leaving me to spend another year in school and try again the following year. I had to say goodbye to the friends I'd spent three years with and adjust my script regarding when I would graduate, which changed my timeline for getting married and getting on with my life. I was in my twenties, so a year seemed like a *very long* time.

So what happened during that "lost" year? I sought practicum experiences outside of my program and got hooked into the sleep medicine world, which opened up a new career direction I had no idea existed. I made two new friends, who became two of my best friends, and I got to spend a year hanging out with them. I had the opportunity to spend more time with my best friend in the year before she got married. All in all, that "lost" year was one of my most fun ones in graduate school. Even better, I found a career path I love.

What Doesn't Kill You . . .

We've all heard the phrase, "What doesn't kill you makes you stronger." Of course the internet disagrees, and I don't want to negate anyone's trauma, but often what the overachiever fears is missing out on some great opportunity. We invented FOMO (fear of missing out) before it was a thing.

The biggest problem with this fear of missing opportunities is that it can cause the phenomenon of "analysis paralysis." Yes, I'm hitting all the meme phrases in this section. Please pass the cat pictures and avocados. But think about opportunity FOMO, which could also be thought of as fear of setbacks: It can prevent a person from making any decision. "I just don't know what to do," my clients will tell me. "How do I choose?"

First challenge the idea that a wrong choice will ruin your life. I've seen this belief in many of my younger patients. One who faced a decision of what department in their company to join expressed the concern that if they chose wrong, it could derail their entire career. Chances are that won't happen. Sure, it could potentially delay things by a few years, but even then, it's a learning experience.

Another client in that age group expressed frustration that their chance for advancement had been sabotaged, and so they wouldn't make manager when the others who had joined the company around the same time did. I agreed with their frustration, but I encouraged them to try to see other opportunities and widen their focus. Career setbacks, although they feel horrible, are unlikely to derail one's entire career trajectory.

I have a wise friend who once said an interesting phrase that I sometimes repeat to myself. "Is it going to end up with you dead, committed, or in jail? If not, then it's probably okay."

And who knows? Making the "wrong" decision now could lead to better things in the future.

We're All Unfinished Works

When do you know you've made it, that you've arrived? When you're making a lot of money? When your kids are doing well in school? When you own your dream house? When you can retire comfortably, or more than comfortably?

Everyone has a different measure of success. The problem – and the joy of it – for the overachiever is that we're never quite there. We may accomplish one thing, but we don't take the time to celebrate it before moving on to the next task, the next hurdle. But what happens when we run out of things to jump over?

Overachievers do not simply coast.

As I mentioned previously, I see this situation as the midlife crisis for someone with our personality type. Again, we have the opportunity to treat the lack of giant goal-targets as a challenge. Perhaps it's time to work on something more important or meaningful to you. For example, I can say from experience that achieving and maintaining one's health can be an ongoing project. One evening at the gym I said to my friend Hank (who doesn't remember this conversation), "When do I get to the point where I don't have to exercise or worry about what I eat?"

"Anne," he replied, "I believe that's called death."

The point is, we've all got something to improve upon. But is it meaningful enough for us to pursue it?

Preparing for setbacks

If setbacks are inevitable, can we prepare for them?

My thought is yes. I'm not suggesting you engage in the "hope for the best and prepare for the worst" attitude. That's pessimism in disguise. Rather, practice doing something that we overachievers hate – being bad at something.

Remember those values I mentioned in the relaxation chapter? One of mine is meaningful connections with others, which means I sometimes end up in situations I wouldn't have otherwise volunteered for. I also value having a range of experiences. That's how I ended up taking belly dancing classes, something I never thought I'd do.

Like many women, I took dance classes as a child. When I asked my mother why I didn't continue with ballet, she said that the teacher moved me into a class that was more advanced than I was prepared for, so I got frustrated and wanted to stop. And my parents let me. I'm guessing this is a common scenario for many overachievers – we didn't persist in activities we weren't good at unless we enjoyed them, but part of the enjoyment is being good at something. All that is to say, I don't have a background in dance, and I'm pretty uncoordinated.

So back to the belly dance classes. My best friend had started dancing at a studio about halfway between our houses (we live about 25 miles apart), and she invited me to join her. I said sure, why not? I'd get to hang out with her, get a good workout, and maybe learn a thing or two I can use in my writing in the future. That's another motivator for me – I never know when a random piece of knowledge may come in handy.

We started with beginner's classes. What to do with your hips, arms, legs — and how to move them all at the same time in different directions. I got exposed to music I would never have listened to otherwise, and I danced to songs from places I'd only seen the names of in books.

The best part, beyond all the cool learning and the fact that every class was a great workout? I wasn't good at it, and it was okay. I remember the moment I realized how much fun I was having precisely because I didn't have to be good at it. It was during the introduction to one dance – by then we'd progressed from basics to choreographed numbers – and I couldn't do the head slide move. My neck muscles just don't work like that. But it didn't matter. I wasn't there to prove anything, and I could have fun in the moment.

Part of the reason I could enjoy myself was that I could separate the activity of belly dancing from the need to perform well. I'd decided not to be in any studio recitals, more because I didn't want to shimmy and shake my bare belly in front of an audience that may contain a past or current client. There are some contexts you should never see your therapist in. But if I was aiming to perform, I'd have to feel competent, and I didn't. I didn't need to show what I could do to anyone except my teachers, who had a great balance of understanding for us amateurs and the ability to push us when needed.

My friend, who has a much more extensive dance background and who was good at belly dancing, did perform, and I went to cheer her on. We stopped dancing when she got pregnant with her third child and I got my third book contract. In other words, life got in the way. But I'll never forget the lessons from that time: do something just for fun, not because you want to be good at it – and it's okay to not be good at something, right away or ever.

So how can you stretch yourself to practice not being good at something?

Conclusion: Celebrate Setbacks

I'd never planned to be a sleep psychologist in private practice, but if I'd "succeeded" at matching to internship that first time, I would have missed out on what has been an amazing career, and I probably would have been miserable in academia. I would also have lost the opportunity to make and solidify some of my most important friendships.

It takes the perspective of time and age to realize that

setbacks often turn into the opportunities that define our life directions. So, getting back to my current script change, while I don't get to be a mother, I'm sure I'll have opportunities for other cool and interesting life stuff. Like writing this book, which may have never happened otherwise.

Important Takeaways

- Setbacks are inevitable. The difference between the amateur and the professional is how you handle them.
- There's no way to know what will happen in life and work. Making the "wrong" decision can lead to better opportunities in the future.
- Practicing something for fun and values, even if you're not good at it, can be fulfilling in other ways.
- Script changes happen. While it can be difficult to recognize them as opportunities, often they can be important and beneficial turning points.

PROCRASTINATION – IT'S THE LAST CHAPTER FOR A REASON

A couple of weeks before I finished this book I went down the most ironic research rabbit hole – I got caught up in downloading and printing out articles on procrastination. I recognized this and confessed it to my office manager, who observed me going back and forth between my office and the large printer in the front office closet.

"I'm printing off articles on procrastination," I told her. "It's the last chapter in my book, and I'm caught up in researching it."

She came back with a pithy and wise comment, as she typically does: "Write what you know, right?"

While the research says that 20–25 percent of the population has trouble with procrastination, and that number is as high as 70 percent in university students (surprise)[1], I have found it to be one of my overachieving clients' most consistent complaints. Often it comes out as a combination of a lamentation and confession: "Why can't I make myself do__?"

Plus – you guessed it – what do some sleep-interfering thoughts consist of? Unfinished tasks and the negative judgments about ourselves that come with them. Another way procrastination interferes with sleep, as we'll talk about later, is that those tasks have to be done sometime, and so they can eat into our sleep opportunity.

Perfectionism and Procrastination: Kissing Cousins

As I mentioned in chapter six, perfectionism is one reason we put things off. We're afraid of failing, and if we don't feel as if we're good at something, we avoid it. This happens especially when we feel like we're going to be judged. That's why writing this book took me over three years, whereas my novels take me three to six months total, if I were to add up the time.

By the way, fellow writers, this is the length of time it *currently* takes me to write a novella or novel. I've written sixteen of them at this point. It used to take me much longer.

With my fiction, I can also hide behind my pen name and the associated persona. This book? It's me, Anne Bartolucci, psychologist and overachiever, standing in front of you, hoping you'll like me and my book (brownie points if you can tell what movie I'm misquoting).

What Is Procrastination?

When you start studying psychology, one thing that becomes clear is that no one can agree on the definition of anything. Or, as one psychologist I interviewed for my *Business Basics for Private Practice* book said, "Put ten psychologists in a room, and you'll get fifteen different opinions."

I like to joke that when they do research, psychologists set out to prove what everyone knows already. My dissertation was on sleep deprivation, irritability, and aggression. Yeah, duh. That said, I've never felt threatened by one of my insomnia clients. Most of them are too tired to do anything aggressive.

Had I continued in academia, I would have likely gone into the aggression/personality/sleep field. I would also have struggled to publish, because I found the satisfaction in figuring out stuff, not in sharing it. My feeling was, "okay, figured it out, let's move on." Plus academic writing is *bo-ring* and not my style. All that passive voice – ick. And there's really no plot.

How much did I struggle with formal academic style? My graduate advisor rejected the first draft of my dissertation because he said it was written in too entertaining a style. I wish I'd realized then that it pointed me to a different calling. My first fiction book wouldn't be published until about nine years later.

Right, back to procrastination. The current (mostly) agreed-upon definition is that procrastination is putting off something that one needs to do but that has negative consequences for avoiding. If you want the true academic definition from an honest-to-goodness procrastination researcher, here you go: "The voluntary delay of an intended and necessary and/or [personally] important activity, despite expecting potential negative consequences that outweigh the positive consequences of the delay."[2]

When I was talking about this chapter with one of my patients, they told me that sometimes their procrastination had been rewarded because whatever they'd been avoiding ended up either being taken care of or no longer an issue. According to the definition, that's not true procrastination. Neither is waiting to get a printer cartridge until I had a coupon, which is what I did recently, although it felt like I was putting it off.

What about my procrastinating writing this book for a long time? The action did have negative consequences – I felt badly about myself. And I felt that I needed to do it, but it's not as if I had a book contract or a deadline. I wouldn't have to pay back an advance or otherwise be penalized. The only issue was that I would disappoint the people who'd been looking forward to it.

That made it personally meaningful, and I hope this book will help me professionally as well.

Perhaps this is where the definition of procrastination falls short for overachievers. We put a lot of pressure on ourselves, and whereas there may not be any *external* negative consequences, we have a lot of internal ones. In short, we're good at beating ourselves up for it. But that doesn't help, as we'll see.

What Do We Procrastinate?

As with much of psychological research, the bulk of the procrastination literature comes out of studies of undergraduate students. They're nice captive research participants. Another one of my jokes is that my dissertation was an animal study – all my subjects were undergraduate males. Okay, that's not fair, but it usually gets a laugh from my audience, especially from the parents of undergraduate males. I did find one study that attempted to look beyond that population. Sorry, the researchers looked beyond that population. See? Academic writing. It tries to pull you in.

The study[3] looked at six domains of life and found that people are most likely to procrastinate in three of them: work/school, medical, and "everyday obligations," or things we have to do but that aren't work- or school-related. Guess what I hear about most during the spring? Yep, taxes. What do people procrastinate less on? Leisure, family/partnership, and social contacts.

Here's a great example of psychology proving things we already know – we're less likely to put off what we enjoy (leisure) or what's meaningful to us (family and partnership). Social contacts could fall under either.

The review paper I looked at[2] listed several types of tasks that people tend to procrastinate on. Things that are unpleasant, difficult, or not appealing tend to be put off, as do assignments we don't believe we can get done. We also procrastinate things that have a far-off rather than a more immediate reward or, I suspect, consequence. That fits in with the health-related procrastination mentioned previously.

Finally, some researchers have speculated that there are different types of procrastination. Arousal/approach procrastination is the type where people put stuff off until there's a deadline, because they get a rush from the challenge of trying to meet it. The other type, which is the one most of us are familiar with, is avoidance procrastination. That occurs when we delay doing something so that if it turns out badly, we can blame the time crunch rather than our lack of ability. Avoidance procrastination also comes out of anxiety, as we'll see in the next section.

Why Do We Procrastinate?

This is where the research gets interesting, and thankfully there was a review paper that laid out all this information nicely so I didn't have to go look for it myself[2]. The reasons for procrastination range from it being tied to one or more personality traits, including perfectionism, to a failure in motivation, which I'm not sure I buy for my overachievers, to environmental factors.

When it comes to personality, one interesting tie-in to the overachiever personality is that people with cluster c personality disorders, such as obsessive-compulsive personality disorder, are more inclined to procrastinate. If you think about it, wanting to have everything "just so" and knowing how unlikely that is to happen could produce a mental block due to fear of failing. But the flip side of this is that not completing a task ensures failure, which leads the procrastinator to feel worse about themselves.

Boredom and procrastination also tend to occur together.

This is particularly true for those who have been diagnosed with ADHD, although not necessarily for those who have some ADHD characteristics but don't meet the full criteria. When I do my talk on procrastination, I discuss boredom and its definition, which is tied to high levels of emotion, difficulty with focus, and lack of situational control[1].

It's funny how control keeps coming up. Isn't that one reason why we engage in perfectionism – the bargains we try to make to ensure our happiness?

As you've probably guessed by now, the way we think affects what we do and how we feel. One hypothesis that repeatedly comes up in the Rational-Emotive Behavioral Therapy (REBT) realm is that procrastination is the way people protect their sense of self worth. In other words, doing well on a task means that one is worthy, and on the other side, failure means they're an awful person. Sound familiar? Check this out: "absolutistic and rigid demands (doing well at almost anything, getting approval from others, having comfortable life situations and being treated fairly by others) contribute to procrastination."[4]

They may as well have said, "being an overachiever makes you likely to procrastinate." These authors went on to demonstrate that self-doubt led to fear of failure in the presence of high levels of irrational beliefs, such as self-criticism, craving the positive opinion of others, and the desire to complete tasks. Participants who had high levels of rational beliefs – more logical, objective views of situations – were less likely to procrastinate, even if they feared failure. They put it all together by showing that self-doubt works through fear of failure to increase the likelihood of procrastination.

The Problem with "Laziness"

As I mentioned in the section above, procrastinators tend to judge themselves negatively, and doing so increases the likelihood of the behavior itself. One term I often hear from my overachiever clients is *lazy*, as in, "I'm so lazy, I don't know why I can't get this thing done." They attribute their failure to a dispositional trait – laziness – rather than a situational one or even a cognitive one.

What is laziness? Those of us who remember the Smurfs may recall Lazy Smurf, who slept all the time. I bet he had a sleep disorder, but "Sleep Apnea Smurf" or "Narcoleptic Smurf" just doesn't have the same ring to it. The poor little guy just couldn't stay awake, and therefore he couldn't really do much. That's how my overachiever patients see themselves – as unable to accomplish what they want. And they beat themselves up over it because they think it's because they don't care enough to overcome whatever is getting in their way. Therefore, they must be lazy.

I would argue that rather than procrastinating because they don't care enough, these "lazy" people care too much, but about the wrong things. Remember, the need for approval runs high in overachieving individuals. So does the need for accomplishment, which could be reworded as the desire for a good outcome. But how often do outcomes fall completely under our control? Rarely. We can control what we do to a point, and we can try to set up circumstances for success, but in the end, there's always the element of luck or chance. I can do everything I think I'm supposed to do for a book release, and the book could still flop. I can follow all the clinical guidelines and my own experience and still not help someone sleep well. Thankfully this occurs rarely. I can prepare for a difficult conversation, use all my magical psychology communication tools, and still not get the outcome I want.

The scary thing is, we're not in as much control as we like to think we are. At certain points in our lives, this truth rears its ugly head. We tend to defend ourselves through procrastination, because otherwise we'd blame ourselves for the lack of outcomes we can't guarantee.

Procrastination and Sleep

As with many psychological variables, procrastination and sleep difficulties make for an interesting chicken-and-egg question. We know that poor sleep leads to increased procrastination, especially when the hours you sleep are not the ones your body wants you to[5]. Studies have also shown that procrastination predicts sleep problems[6], and that those whose clocks are set later are more likely to procrastinate.

Through the years, I've noticed an interesting phenomenon with my overachieving clients: bedtime procrastination. I didn't realize until I started researching this section that this specific type of procrastination behavior was so common.

Bedtime procrastination, as the name implies, is putting off getting in bed, and therefore robbing oneself of adequate amounts of sleep. Why does this occur? Some authors have posited that people find their prebedtime routine to be aversive in some way[7]. I find, however, that many of my clients like their prebedtime routines but get caught up in the "one more thing" trap – that is, *I need to do just one more thing before I start heading to bed*.

Like other types of procrastination, putting off starting the prebedtime routine can be thought of as failure of some self-control process, which can also be thought of as self-regulation. In other words, when I'm faced with something appealing or something aversive, can I control my thoughts, behaviors, and emotions? Or do I give in to whatever my mind and body want my first response to be?

Of course beliefs play a part, too. Do I believe that I lack discipline or willpower? If so, I'm more likely to procrastinate. But overachievers can be disciplined people. Perhaps the issue is that we believe willpower is something we only have a certain amount of. One study found that after days rated as stressful, participants delayed bedtime unnecessarily if they believed in willpower as a limited resource, but not if they believe it's something people don't run out of[7].

Overcoming Procrastination

I once saw a comic that simply portrayed a sign that said something like, "Procrastinators Anonymous, Meeting Postponed." What do you do about a process that is associated with delaying rather than taking action?

Self-efficacy, or the belief that you can accomplish something, is one theme that arises over and over in the procrastination literature. One thing that has helped my overachieving clients is to focus on one part of the task, the first step. Completing an entire project or losing five pounds can be intimidating to think about, but taking one small step toward those goals – gathering resources or changing one dietary habit – can nudge someone along. The step also has to be something you feel willing and able to do. For example, you may not be willing to make a phone call to someone, but how about an email? Or you might not want to give up your bedtime snack, but you could change it from ice cream to fruit so you still satisfy your sugar habit.

Another strategy has been to modify beliefs. Realistically, what is the worst thing that could result from you not doing as well at something as you want to or believe you should? Also, think of the relief you'll feel when you're finally done with whatever you've been avoiding.

As you'll probably not be surprised to read, mindfulness

has been found to protect against procrastination tendencies[8], and it can help reduce the effects of procrastination on stress and health[9]. One theory is that part of the reason people put off tasks is due to the negative thoughts about them and then the negative thoughts about not completing the tasks. This creates a vicious cycle, because then the person's energy goes into beating themselves up rather than finishing the task. Mindfulness can help us step out of this cycle by looking at the thoughts nonjudgmentally and stepping back from them rather than struggling with them[9].

Part of mindfulness is values, and when we're engaged in value-related activities, we're less likely to procrastinate. Sometimes it takes a little more effort to find the value in certain activities than it does with others. The concept of elements of interest from the ADHD world may be helpful. If someone is faced with a task they perceive as aversive and/or boring, finding something interesting about it can be motivating[10]. For example, many writers hate marketing. I got over that by figuring out that it satisfies my desire to do research and see what happens when I manipulate variables.

It can also be helpful to know what else motivates you – for good or bad. For example, one of the things that motivated me to leap into private practice was fear of missing out on the opportunity to join the space-sharing arrangement I started out in. I partially attribute that decision to my gut telling me it was time, but good ol' FOMO gave me the push. The same occurred with this book. The nonfiction editor I'd contracted with started a job, and I knew her time might become more limited, so I didn't want to miss out on the opportunity to work with her.

It can also be useful to examine one's beliefs about oneself. I've had several patients who were convinced that deadlines motivate them, and that's the only way they can accomplish tasks. However, their stress levels rose and their sleep quality plummeted when it was "crunch time." Behavioral experiments – seeing what results from doing something differently, for good or ill – could be helpful.

In mindfulness, nothing is all good or all bad, even perfectionism. Although perfectionism can lead to procrastination, parts of it can protect against it. One study defined something called "adaptive perfectionism," or the useful parts, specifically having high standards for oneself and being organized and goal-oriented. If you can use mindfulness or some other technique to separate those bits from the self-doubt and fear of making mistakes, you can use those perfectionistic tendencies to overcome procrastination[11].

In other words, you can use your overachiever tendencies to overcome procrastination. On the flip side, you can also use procrastination to deal with itself in a method called structured procrastination, which entails getting something done by using it to procrastinate doing something else that also needs to be done. It sounds like a lot of mental gymnastics, but it's not that bad. *The Art of Procrastination* by John Perry[12] is a good resource if you'd like to try this strategy.

IF YOU TAKE anything from this chapter, hopefully it's a strategy or two to try, but also the message that you don't need to beat yourself up for procrastinating. It's a human tendency. Digging deeper into the why and challenging the maladaptive beliefs at the heart of it can be the first step to overcoming it, but sometimes, as the Nike brand slogan says, you need to Just Do It. Or maybe the first step.

Important Takeaways

- Procrastination involves avoiding tasks in such a way

that you end up experiencing negative consequences for not getting whatever it was done. Often, for overachievers, these negative consequences are internal.

- People procrastinate for different reasons, for example, out of perfectionism or boredom. Knowing why you procrastinate – and what motivates you to take the first step on something – can help you overcome your blocks.

- Mindfulness can be a useful strategy in overcoming procrastination tendencies.

- Overachiever tendencies combined with structured procrastination can help you to move forward.

10

FINAL THOUGHTS

Dear fellow overachiever, thank you for sticking with me through this journey. I hope you've found some helpful tips and tricks. More importantly, my wish for you is that you've learned some things that will help you to be more compassionate toward yourself. That's one of the few ways "why" questions are useful — they help us acknowledge and better deal with why we do things and to accept our humanity and the processes it entails. Yes, we can always do better. Yes, it can take time to figure out how, and that's okay.

Am I perfect? No. Do I still make some of the mistakes I discuss in this book? Definitely. I still sleep great, though.

One way procrastination bit me in the butt with this project was that I delayed its release right into a pandemic. However, I still believe in looking for the hope in what could be a setback, so perhaps this book is timely because you know what, fellow overachievers?

Situations like this are hell for us, and we can use all the support we can get. Our goals have been stalled, perhaps some of you have lost incomes or even jobs, and we're all dealing with more uncertainty than our minds could have possibly imagined. Ugh, uncertainty sucks, doesn't it? It means we can't do what we do best — plan and prepare. Plus we have that visceral fear response to something we can't see that potentially wants to kill us, so the situation is hitting us at the deepest core of our survival instincts. Being in survival mode dings our ability to focus and be productive because we don't have all our usual mental resources at our disposal.

On the other hand, one of the ways we overachievers thrive is through finding opportunity, even if it's to work on ourselves. That's why I'm happy you picked up this book, especially now. I've found myself fortunate to continue working – psychologists are busy right now – and I've also had to figure out what truths, both pleasant and unpleasant, I need to learn. One of them is that I've gotten so caught up in my practice and writing bubbles that I've neglected some of the things that are most important to me.

As you've read throughout this book, you have hopefully seen that being an overachiever can be a double-edged sword. It helps us to accomplish great things. It also can keep us from feeling good about them and make us focus too much on the future. Right now, as it's nearly impossible to plan for the future, being more in the present and cherishing our everyday moments of delight is a necessary practice not only for peace, but for mental survival.

When I was in college, I came to the realization that if I were to ponder the uncertainty inherent in life, I would put myself into an anxious state. I was probably taking philosophy at the time. I recognized on some level that we're in control of very little, and it can be paralyzing to think about what *could* happen. Yes, this has definitely been more on my mind recently.

However, now that I've achieved a couple more decades of maturity, I've come to see the freedom in uncertainty. Sure, I may not be able to control everything, but that also opens up the space for fun and interesting things to happen. Or bad things – but typically the surprises in my life have been good. As long as I've stuck to my values and opened myself to opportunities, I've found more joy than I would have thought possible and had experiences I never could have imagined.

So, dear fellow overachiever, I first commend you for everything you've accomplished, and I hope you'll take a moment to give yourself some credit for those things as well. Second, again, I hope that if nothing else, this book has led you to self-compassion and yes, to better sleep through healthier habits and understanding. If you continue to learn from the past, plan for but not obsess about the future, and live according to your values, there's a good chance peace will follow, even when life isn't perfect.

I do hope you'll share your thoughts and feedback with me either at my website overachieverbook.com or through the email list (https://overachieverbook.com/newsletter). I'll continue to read and review resources you may find useful that pertain to the topics covered in this book.

I WISH you many adventures and yes, much achievement, whatever that looks like for you.

FINAL FINAL THOUGHT:

Reviews are tremendously important and help other readers find books. If you found Better Sleep for the Overachiever to be useful - or even if you didn't - it would be amazing if you could leave a review at the site where you bought the book. Thank you!

ABOUT DR. BARTOLUCCI

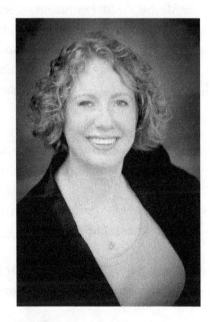

Anne Bartolucci, Ph.D., C.B.S.M. is a licensed psychologist and
a certified behavioral sleep medicine specialist. She started her
professional career as the clinical director of a sleep disorders
center and founded Atlanta Insomnia & Behavioral Health

Services, P.C. in 2008 in order to focus specifically on behavioral treatment for sleep disorders. At any one time, approximately 80-90% of her caseload time consists of patients with insomnia.

Dr. Bartolucci is a sought-after speaker and conference panelist and has taught workshops and classes for several organizations such as the American Academy of Dental Sleep Medicine, the Atlanta School of Sleep Medicine, the Anxiety and Stress Management Institute, and the Georgia Psychological Association. She is also adjunct faculty at Emory University and lectures to the sleep and psychiatry fellows. She is the author of two nonfiction books - *Business Basics for Private Practice: A Guide for Mental Health Practitioners* (2017; Routledge) and *Better Sleep for the Overachiever*, which is slated for a September 2020 release. Finally, she has a not-so-secret other life as a U.S.A. Today bestselling fiction author under the pen name Cecilia Dominic, and sleep and its mysteries keep sneaking into her storylines.

You can find her and information about how to book her as a speaker on her practice website: https://sleepyintheatl.com

She also blogs about her own experiences as an overachiever at: https://overachieverbook.com

If you'd like more sleep tips, please sign up for her email newsletter at: https://overachieverbook.com/newsletter

Finally, if you're interested in reading her fiction books, including the Dream Weavers & Truth Seekers series mentioned in the book, please go to https://ceciliadominic.com

APPENDIX: REFERENCES AND NOTES

Chapter One: You might be an overachiever if...
[1] T. J. Delong. (2011). *Flying without a Net: Turn Fear of Change into Fuel for Success.* Boston: Harvard Business Review.

Chapter Two: Why is this happening to me?
[1] A. J. Spielman, L. S. Caruso, and P. B. Glovinsky. 1987. "A Behavioral Perspective on Insomnia Treatment." *Psychiatric Clinics of North America* 10: 541–553.
[2] R. R. McRae and P. T. Costa. 1987. "Validation of the Five-Factor Model of Personality across Instruments and Observers." *Journal of Personality and Social Psychology* 52: 81–90.
[3] E. K. Gray and D. Watson. 2002. "General and Specific Traits of Personality and Their Relation to Sleep and Academic Performance." *Journal of Personality* 70: 177–206.
[4] H-N. Kim, et al. 2015. "Association between Personality Traits and Sleep Quality in Young Korean Women." *PLoS ONE* 10, no. 6: e0129599. doi:10.137/journal.pone.0129599.
[5] M. Hintsanen, et al. 2014. "Five-Factor Personality Traits and Sleep: Evidence from Two Population-Based Cohort Studies." *Health Psychology* 33: 1214–1233.

[6] M. J. Boudreaux. 2016. "Personality-Related Problems and the Five-Factor Model of Personality." *Personality Disorders: Theory, Research, and Treatment*, March 28, advance online publication. http://dx.doi.org/10.1037/per0000185.

[7] M. Van de Laar, et al. 2010. "The Role of Personality Traits in Insomnia." *Sleep Medicine Reviews* 14: 61–68.

[8] American Psychiatric Association. 2013. *Diagnostic and Statistical Manual of Mental Disorders* (*DSM-5*). Washington, D.C: American Psychiatric Association.

[9] Reference pending.

[10] S. A. Sassoon, et al. 2014. "Association between Personality Traits and DSM-IV Diagnosis of Insomnia in Perimenopausal Women: Insomnia and Personality in Perimenopause." *Menopause* 21, no. 6: 602–611.

[10] M. E. Ruiter, et al. 2012. "Personality Disorder Features and Insomnia Status amongst Hypnotic-Dependent Adults." *Sleep Medicine* 13: 1122–1129.

[11] S. Coren. 1988. "Prediction of Insomnia from Arousability Predisposition Score: Scale Development and Crossvalidation." *Behaviour Research and Therapy* 26: 415–420.

[12] J. Fernandez-Mendoza, et al. 2010. "Cognitive-Emotional Hyperarousal as a Premorbid Characteristic of Individuals Vulnerable to Insomnia." *Psychosomatic Medicine* 72: 397–403.

[13] M. LeBlanc, et al. 2009. "Incidence and Risk Factors of Insomnia in a Population-Based Sample." *SLEEP* 32, no. 8: 1027–1037.

[14] C. M. Morin, S. Rodrigue, and H. Ivers. 2003. "Role of Stress, Arousal, and Coping Skills in Primary Insomnia." *Psychosomatic Medicine* 65: 259–267.

[15] C. J. Harvey, P. Gehrman, and C. A. Espie. 2014. "Who is Predisposed to Insomnia: A Review of Familial Aggregation, Stress-Reactivity, Personality and Coping Style." *Sleep Medicine Reviews* 18: 237–247.

[16] Reference pending.

Chapter Three: Busting sleep myths

[1] Hung, et al. 2018 "Risk of Dementia in Patients with Primary Insomnia: A Nationwide Population-Based Case-Control Study." *BMC Psychiatry* 18, article 38. https://doi.org/10.1186/s12888-018-1623-0.

[2] K.G. Baron, S. Abbott, N. Jao, N. Manalo, R. Mullen. 2017. "Orthosomnia: Are Some Patients Taking the Quantified Self Too Far?" *Journal of Clinical Sleep Medicine* 13, no. 2: 351–354.

[3] R. Ekirch. 2006. *At Day's Close: Night in Times Past.* New York: Norton.

[4] M.A. Carskadon and W.C. Dement 2011. "Normal Human Sleep: An Overview." In *Principles and Practice of Sleep Medicine*, 5th edition, edited by M.H. Kryger, T. Roth, and W.C. Dement, 16–26. St. Louis: Elsevier Saunders.

[5] C. Depner et al. (2019). "Ad Libitum Weekend Recovery Sleep Fails to Prevent Metabolic Dysregulation during a Repeating Pattern of Insufficient Sleep and Weekend Recovery Sleep." *Current Biology* 29: 1. doi: 10.1016/j.cub.2019.01.069.

Chapter Four: Relaxation for those who can't relax

[1] L. Roember and S. M. Orsillo. 2009. *Mindfulness and Acceptance-Based Therapies in Practice.* New York: Guilford.

[2] S.C. Hayes, K.D. Strosahl, and K.G. Wilson. 1999. *Acceptance and Commitment Therapy: An Experiential Approach to Behavior Change.* New York: Guilford.

[3] N. Quenk 1993. *Beside Ourselves: Our Hidden Personality in Everyday Life.* Palo Alto: Davies Black Publishing. p. 143.

Note: While looking for references for the diaphragmatic breathing, I found it's one of those things that people know works, but its origins are muddy. When I searched for references I found in other places, I found that the journal databases I had access to did not have the journals or articles I needed. Many people cite The Relaxation Response, a book that brought Transcendental Meditation into the relaxation sphere in the 1970s. Admittedly, I've never read it, although one of my clients kept threatening to give me a copy. Across the research, it's evident that diaphragmatic breathing has been shown to be beneficial for stress and physiological arousal.

Chapter Five: Sleep smarter, or what to do about your racing mind

[1] L. Roember and S. M. Orsillo. 2009. *Mindfulness and Acceptance-Based Therapies in Practice.* New York: Guilford.

[2] S.C. Hayes, K.D. Strosahl, and K.G. Wilson. 1999. *Acceptance and Commitment Therapy: An Experiential Approach to Behavior Change.* New York: Guilford.

[3] D. Altman. 2014. *The Mindfulness Toolbox: Fifty Practical Tips, Tools, and Handouts for Anxiety, Depression, Stress, and Pain.* Eau Claire, Wisconsin: Pesi.

[4] J. Beck. 1995. *Cognitive Therapy: Basics and Beyond.* New York: Guilford.

[5] D. Greenberger, & C. A. Padesky. 2016. Mind over mood: Change how you feel by changing the way you think (2nd ed.). New York: Guilford.

[6] S. M. Orsillo & L. Roemer. 2011. The mindful way through anxiety: Break free from worry and reclaim your life. New York: Guilford.

Chapter Six: Perfectionism

[1] S. Nicely and R. Wilson. 2018. *Is Fred in the Refrigerator?: Taming OCD and Reclaiming My Life.* Atlanta: Nicely Done Publishing.

[2] T. Åkerstedt, F. Ghilotti, A. Grotta, et al. 2019. "Sleep Duration and Mortality: Does Weekend Sleep Matter?" *Journal of Sleep Research* 28: e12712. DOI: 10.1111/jsr.12712

[3] M. Breus. 2016. *The Power of When: Discover Your Chronotype – And the Best Time to Eat Lunch, Ask for a Raise, Have Sex,*

Write a Novel, Take Your Meds, and More. New York: Little, Brown.

[4] M. McArdle. February 12, 2014. "Why Writers Are the Worst Procrastinators: The Psychological Origins of Waiting (. . . and Waiting, and Waiting) to Work." *The Atlantic.* (www.theatlantic.com/business/archive/2014/02/why-writers-are-the-worst-procrastinators/283773/)

Chapter Seven: Time management

[1] S. R. Covey. 1989. *The Seven Habits of Highly Effective People: Restoring the Character Ethic.* New York: Simon and Schuster.

[2] D. Allen. 2001. *Getting Things Done: The Art of Stress-Free Productivity.* New York:Viking.

[3] J. Penn. 2016. *The Successful Author Mindset: A Handbook for Surviving the Writer's Journey.* CreateSpace.

[4] A. Bartolucci. 2017. *Business basics for private practice: A guide for mental health professionals.* New York: Routledge.

[5] A. Lakein. 1989. *How to Get Control of Your Time and Your Life.* New York: Dutton.

[6] C. Carney and W.F. Waters. 2006. "Effects of a Structured Problem-Solving Procedure on Pre-Sleep Cognitive Arousal in College Students with Insomnia." *Behavioral Sleep Medicine* 4, no. 1: 13–28.

Chapter Eight: Handling the inevitable – failures and setbacks

This one comes from my life experience, so no references. Don't worry, the next chapter has a lot of research behind it.

Funny story – when I told my father that I was taking belly dance classes, he thought I said, "ballet dance." I never corrected him. It will be interesting to see if he says anything after reading this book. Update - he didn't.

By the way, the studio my friend and I went to closed, and our favorite teacher left, so we never got back to belly dancing. It's a bummer because that was a REALLY good ab workout.

No, I still can't slide my head horizontally. I'll never walk like an Egyptian. Oh, well.

Chapter nine: Procrastination – it's the last chapter for a reason

[1] S. Shellenbarger. January 7, 2014. "To Stop Procrastinating, Look to the Science of Mood Repair. *The Wall Street Journal.* online.wsj.com/news/ articles/SB10001424052702303933104579306664120892036

[2] K.B. Klingsieck. 2013a. "Procrastination: When Good Things Don't Come to Those Who Wait." *European Psychologist* 18, no. 1: 24–34.

[3] K.B. Klingsieck. 2013b. "Procrastination in Different Life Domains: Is Procrastination Domain Specific?" *Current Psychology* 32: 175–185.

[4] M. Balkis and E. Duru. 2019. "Procrastination and Rational/Irrational Beliefs: A Moderated Mediation Model." *Journal of Rational-Emotive and Cognitive-Behavioral Therapy* 37: 299–315. https://doi.org/10.1007/s10942-019-00314-6.

[5] J. Kühnel, S. Sonnentag, R. Bledow, and K.G. Melchers. 2018. The Relevance of Sleep and Circadian Misalignment for Procrastination among Shift Workers. *Journal of Occupational and Organizational Psychology* 91: 110–133.

[6] A. Przepiórka, A. Blachnio, and N.Y.F. Siu. 2019. "The Relationships between Self-Efficacy, Self-Control, Chronotype, Procrastination and Sleep Problems in Young Adults." *Chronobiology International* 6: 1025–1035.

[7] K. Bernecker and V. Job. 2019. "Too Exhausted to Go to Bed: Implicit Theories about Willpower and Stress Predict Bedtime Procrastination." *British Journal of Psychology.* https://doi.org/10.1111/bjop.12382.

[8] R.Y.M. Cheung and M.C.Y. Ng. 2019. "Being in the Moment Later? Testing the Inverse Relation between Mindfulness and Procrastination." *Personality and Individual Differences* 141: 123–126.

[9] F.M. Sirois and N. Tosti. 2012. "Lost in the Moment? An Investigation of Procrastination, Mindfulness, and Well-Being. *Journal of Rational-Emotive and Cognitive-Behavior Therapy* 30: 237–248.

[10] L. Sweitzer. 2014. *Beating Boredom as the Secret to Managing ADHD: The Elephant in the ADHD Room.* London: Jessica Kingsley.

[11] A. Burnham, M. Komarraju, R. Hamel, and D.R. Nadler. 2014. "Do Adaptive Perfectionism and Self-Determined Motivation Reduce Academic Procrastination?" *Learning and Individual Differences* 36: 165–172.

[12] Perry, J. (2012). *The Art of Procrastination: A Guide to Effective Dawdling, Lollygagging and Postponing.* New York: Workman.

APPENDIX: SLEEP DIARY

SLEEP DIARY

Unfortunately my pretty image didn't transfer, so please answer the questions below every morning. Don't look at the clock, though. Your best guess is good enough, I promise.

1. Yesterday, I napped from _____ to _____
(note the times of all naps)

2. Yesterday, I took _____ mg of medication
and/or _____ oz of alcohol as a sleep aid.

3. Last night, I went to bed and turned the lights off
at _____ o'clock.

4. After turning the lights out,
I fell asleep in _____ minutes.

5. My sleep was interrupted _____times.
(specify number of nighttime awakenings)

6. My sleep was interrupted for _____ minutes.
(specify duration of each awakening)

7. This morning, I woke up at _____o'clock.
(note time of last awakening when you stayed awake)

8. This morning, I got out of bed at _____o'clock.

(specify the time)

9. When I got up this morning I felt _____

(1 = exhausted, 5 = refreshed)

10. Overall, my sleep last night was _____

(1 = very restless, 5 = very sound)

CPSIA information can be obtained
at www.ICGtesting.com
Printed in the USA
JSHW080414061022
31318JS00002B/99